A Caregiver's Companion

RESILIENCE NAVIGATING GRIEF

Terrie LaRae Harris

Resilience Navigating Grief
A Caregiver's Companion
Terrie LaRae Harris

Contact the author: caregiverscompanion247@gmail.com

Edited by:

Mary Ethel

Mary Ethel Eckard
Frisco, Texas

Library of Congress Control Number: 2025919578
ISBN (Print): 978-1-966561-25-5
ISBN (E-book): 978-1-966561-26-2

CONTENTS

DEDICATION

I dedicate this book to the unsung heroes—the caregivers. To those who tirelessly provide comfort and support, often sacrificing their own well-being in the process. To those who have walked the labyrinthine paths of grief, bearing the weight of loss while simultaneously shouldering the responsibilities of care. Your strength, resilience, and unwavering love inspire us all. May these pages offer solace, understanding, and a path toward healing and renewed hope.

This is for you, the compassionate souls who carry the torch of love even amidst profound sorrow. Your journey is a testament to the enduring power of the human spirit, and this book is a small offering of gratitude and support on your path to healing. May it serve as a quiet companion during the challenging times, offering guidance and validating your experiences. Your dedication to others is a profound gift; may this work serve as a beacon of light, illuminating your path to well-being.

PREFACE

This journey is not just about coping; it's about finding a way forward, even amidst profound sorrow, and discovering a new sense of purpose and well-being. It offers practical strategies and heartfelt insights to help you navigate the complexities of grief, offering comfort and understanding during your darkest moments. I am honored to support and share my experiences to help others navigate grief and heal one heart at a time. This journey is deeply personal, and my hope is that these pages will provide a compassionate companion, guiding you to a future where healing and hope are possible. Through shared experiences and actionable steps, we can find solace and begin to rebuild our lives after loss.

This book guides readers through self-discovery, emphasizing the transformative power of mindfulness and self-care in fostering healing and resilience.

Having endured the agonizing sorrow of losing both parents to cancer, compounded by the devastating death of my eldest child, I understand grief's profound impact intimately. My experiences as a caregiver and my work supporting others in similar situations revealed the intensely personal and uniquely challenging nature of bereavement.

This book, born from a yearning to offer solace and guidance, aims to provide a holistic framework for comprehending the multifaceted aspects of caregiver sorrow. It's not a simplistic prescription for immediate relief, but a compassionate compass guiding readers through self-discovery, emphasizing the transformative power of mindfulness and self-care in fostering healing and resilience. Through a combination of evidence-based therapeutic techniques and moving personal narratives, we will explore the varied emotional responses associated with loss, dismantling common myths and misconceptions surrounding grief.

Understanding that grief is not a linear progression but a fluid, unpredictable journey, I aim to empower readers to validate their feelings, find strength in their vulnerability, and cultivate a nurturing environment for self-care. The exploration of mindfulness and wellness modalities will provide practical tools to cope with the overwhelming emotions that often accompany loss, guiding readers toward a path of resilience and hope.

It is not just about coping; it's about finding a way forward, even amidst profound sorrow, and discovering a new sense of purpose and well-being while navigating grief.

INTRODUCTION

The loss of a loved one is an experience that profoundly alters one's life. For caregivers, this loss is often compounded by the exhaustion and emotional toll of providing care.

We delve into the unique complexities of caregiver grief, recognizing the multifaceted nature of this journey. We'll move beyond the simplistic notion of stages of grief and explore the diverse emotional landscapes individuals must navigate—the intense waves of sadness, anger, guilt, and confusion are an ongoing reality. We'll acknowledge that there is no "right" way to grieve, and that the process is deeply personal and often non-linear.

The chapters that follow will offer an in-depth exploration of grief's multifaceted dimensions. We will delve into the psychological, emotional, and spiritual aspects of loss, providing insights into the various ways individuals cope with bereavement and how these coping mechanisms can impact the healing process. We'll examine the importance of self-compassion, addressing the potential for self-blame and guilt that often surfaces in caregivers. Practical tools and strategies, firmly rooted in evidence-based practices,

We will explore the path of acceptance, not as a destination, but as an ongoing process of integration and healing.

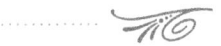

will be introduced. Mindfulness techniques, meditation practices, and other wellness modalities will be presented as valuable resources for navigating overwhelming emotions and fostering a path toward emotional resilience. The focus will remain on empowerment, assisting you in cultivating inner strength, resilience, and hope.

The journey through grief is challenging, but it is not insurmountable. This book provides a framework for understanding, accepting, and navigating the complexities of this emotional landscape, leading you through healing, peace, and a renewed sense of well-being. We will explore the path of acceptance, not as a destination, but as an ongoing process of integration and healing.

Remember, you are not alone on this journey.

CHAPTER 1

The Uniqueness of Caregiver Grief

C aregiver grief is a unique and often intensely challenging experience, distinct from the grief experienced by those who haven't shouldered the responsibilities of caregiving during a loved one's illness or decline. While all grief is deeply personal and unfolds differently for each individual, the added layers of emotional, physical, and logistical burdens faced by caregivers create a particularly complex and demanding journey. Understanding the nuances of caregiver grief is crucial for both caregivers themselves and those who support them.

Understanding the nuances of caregiver grief is crucial for both caregivers themselves and those who support them.

The most immediate distinction lies in the concurrent demands of caregiving and grieving. Imagine a spouse who has diligently cared for their partner battling a long-term illness. The physical and emotional exhaustion from years of providing constant support, coupled with the practicalities of managing medications, appointments, and household tasks, often leaves little room for the caregiver to fully process their own emotional turmoil.

The loss of their partner is not merely a profound emotional blow; it's also the loss of a daily routine, a shared life, and a significant source of emotional connection. The sudden absence of the person who was both the source of their caregiving duties and their primary support network creates a vacuum that leaves many feeling overwhelmed and utterly lost.

This sense of loss is compounded by the often-unseen burden of anticipatory grief. Caregivers frequently experience a prolonged period of grieving before the actual death of their loved one. As the illness progresses, they may start to mentally and emotionally prepare for the inevitable loss, leading to a gradual erosion of their own well-being. This anticipatory grief is often characterized by a profound sense of exhaustion, both physical and emotional. They are already carrying a heavy emotional load while navigating the practicalities of providing constant care; this anticipation only exacerbates their suffering.

Furthermore, the intensity of caregiver grief is often heightened by the experience of guilt. This guilt can manifest in various forms.

Caregivers might grapple with feelings of inadequacy, questioning whether they did enough, provided the best possible care, or made the right decisions throughout the illness. These questions can be especially prevalent when the illness was long and arduous, leading caregivers to scrutinize every aspect of their caregiving approach with agonizing detail. They might feel that their own efforts were insufficient or even that they somehow contributed to their loved one's suffering. This self-blame can significantly intensify the emotional pain and obstruct the grieving process.

The isolation experienced by caregivers is also a critical aspect of their unique grief. While friends and family might offer support, they rarely fully grasp the unique intensity and complexity of their situation. The constant demands of caregiving often lead to social withdrawal, limiting opportunities for social interaction and emotional connection. The inability to participate in activities once enjoyed or to nurture personal relationships adds yet another layer of difficulty. This isolation can create a deep sense of loneliness, exacerbating feelings of hopelessness and despair.

The physical toll of caregiving grief is substantial and often underestimated. The relentless demands of caregiving can lead to sleep deprivation, poor nutrition, and increased stress levels. These factors, combined with the emotional trauma of loss, can significantly impair the caregiver's physical health. They might experience physical ailments, such as chronic pain, digestive problems, or weakened immune systems. The mental strain of navigating grief coupled with the practical challenges of caregiving often leads to a decline in overall health. This physical manifestation of grief reinforces the need for self-care practices to support physical well-being.

These experiences are not unique to a specific demographic. A single mother caring for her terminally ill child will experience this guilt and exhaustion just as profoundly as a spouse caring for a partner with Alzheimer's disease. The common thread is the intensity of the emotional burden combined with the constant demands of caregiving.

> The grieving process for caregivers is often protracted and complex.

The linear stages of grief—denial, anger, bargaining, depression, and acceptance —often fail to capture the intricate reality of their experience. While these stages can provide a framework for understanding grief, they do not account for the fluctuating nature of emotions, the cyclical patterns of grief, and the potential for regressive movements within the process. **A caregiver might feel a sense of relief immediately following the death, only to be overwhelmed by a wave of grief and guilt weeks, months, or**

Acknowledging the unique challenges of caregiver grief is the crucial first step to start healing and finding a new sense of equilibrium.

even years later. This unpredictable and often overwhelming nature of the grieving process makes it particularly important for caregivers to access support and utilize strategies for self-care.

The path toward healing for caregivers necessitates a fundamental shift in perspective. It's not about "getting over" the loss but about learning to live with it. Acknowledging the unique challenges of caregiver grief is the crucial first step to start healing and finding a new sense of equilibrium. **This involves understanding that the emotional rollercoaster of grief is a normal response to an immense loss, and that feelings of guilt, exhaustion, and isolation are not a sign of personal failing but rather a consequence of the intense pressures and emotional burdens involved in caregiving during such a profound loss. Accepting these realities and actively seeking support is crucial to navigating the intricate and emotionally demanding landscape of caregiver grief.** This process requires patience, self-compassion, and a willingness to actively engage in the long road of healing.

The chapters to come will explore specific tools and strategies designed to support caregivers in this journey, empowering them to reclaim their well-being and find a path forward, however long and winding it may be.

CHAPTER 2

Navigating the Stages of Grief

T he common understanding of **grief often portrays a linear progression through distinct stages: denial, anger, bargaining, depression, and acceptance.** While this Kübler-Ross model offers a helpful framework, it's crucial to recognize its limitations.

Grief is not a neat, predictable journey; it's a deeply personal and often chaotic process that unfolds uniquely for each individual. The intensity and order of these emotional responses vary widely, and individuals may experience them repeatedly, out of sequence, or not at all. Expecting a uniform experience can be both unhelpful and invalidating for those struggling with loss.

Let's explore these stages not as rigid boxes, but as potential emotional landscapes one might encounter. **Consider "denial" not as a conscious rejection of reality, but as a temporary buffer against overwhelming pain. It might manifest as a stunned silence, a refusal to believe the news, or a continued engagement in routines as if nothing has changed.** Imagine a caregiver who, after the death of their spouse, continues to set the table for two, instinctively preparing meals and maintaining the household as if their partner is still present. This isn't willful ignorance; it's a coping mechanism, a way to navigate the immediate shock and postpone the full weight of the loss. This phase is temporary, a necessary period of adjustment before the more intense emotions begin to surface.

The **subsequent stage, "anger," often arises as the initial numbness fades. It's not necessarily directed at a specific person or entity; it's a raw expression of the pain, frustration, and injustice of loss.** This anger can manifest in various ways: irritability, resentment, outbursts of rage, or a quiet, simmering bitterness. It may be directed inwards, directed at oneself, fueled by feelings of guilt or inadequacy; or pointed to others, manifesting as impatience, criticism, or withdrawal. A caregiver might direct their anger toward the healthcare system, feeling resentful about the perceived lack of adequate care; they may lash out at family members, expressing their frustration about their own inadequacy, or directing their anger toward a higher power, questioning the fairness of the loss. Understanding this anger as a natural response to pain, rather than a personal failing, is crucial for navigating this emotionally turbulent stage. Be kind to yourself.

"Bargaining," the next stage, often involves attempts to negotiate with a higher power or fate. It's a desperate plea to undo the loss, even if only partially, or to change the circumstances that led to it. This bargaining can be subtle and internal, a silent negotiation with oneself, or more overt, expressed in prayer, promises, or rituals. A caregiver might find themselves bargaining for more time with their loved one, even if only in their memories, replaying past moments and interactions to recapture some of the lost connection. They might bargain for their own well-being, promising to make amends, to be a better person, to live a more fulfilling life, hoping to make a kind of spiritual exchange. These bargains are attempts to regain a sense of control and mitigate the profound helplessness associated with grief.

"Depression," often misinterpreted as simple sadness, is a deeper, more pervasive sense of despair and hopelessness. It's not simply feeling blue; it's a profound sense of emptiness, loss of interest in activities once enjoyed, and a pervasive sense of fatigue. The physical symptoms can be severe: sleep disturbances, appetite changes, and a general lack of energy.

For a caregiver, this depression might be exacerbated by the physical and emotional exhaustion accumulated during the caregiving process. The loss of their loved one not only deprives them of emotional support but also intensifies the burden of managing daily life, leading to further exhaustion and feelings of despair. **Recognizing this depression as a natural response to trauma and not a personal weakness is crucial for seeking appropriate support and intervention.**

Finally, "acceptance" isn't necessarily about feeling happy or "getting over" the loss. It's about gradually integrating the loss into the fabric of one's life, learning to live with the pain, and finding ways to honor the memory of the deceased. This doesn't mean forgetting or ceasing to miss the loved one; instead, it means finding a way to live alongside the grief, to find moments of peace and joy while still acknowledging the enduring sadness.

For a caregiver, acceptance might involve creating rituals to commemorate their loved one, cherishing memories, or **engaging in activities that bring a sense of peace and purpose.** It's about finding a new normal; a life that incorporates both the joy of the past and the challenges of the present.

It's crucial to remember that these stages are not sequential, and their intensity varies significantly. Someone might experience anger intensely before experiencing denial, while another might cycle through these stages repeatedly. Some might experience intense grief initially, then a period of relative calm, only to be hit by waves of intense grief months or years later.

It's this unpredictable nature of grief that highlights the importance of self-compassion and seeking support from others. Grief is not a race to be won; it's a marathon to be navigated, with many ups and downs along the way. The key is to find support, to validate one's feelings, and to allow oneself the time and space needed to heal. This process requires patience, self-compassion, and a willingness to embrace the complexities of grief's unique journey for each individual.

Moreover, the context of caregiver grief adds further layers of complexity. The physical and emotional exhaustion from years of caregiving, the guilt associated with the perceived adequacy of care, and the often-unseen burden of anticipatory grief all significantly shape the emotional landscape. A caregiver might find themselves reliving various stages concurrently, alternating between moments of intense sadness and fleeting glimpses of relief or acceptance. One might experience intense anger at the disease that took their loved one, followed by periods of deep sadness and regret over missed opportunities or unfinished conversations. The lack of a clear-cut linear progression adds to the feeling of disorientation and makes the process even more challenging to navigate.

The variations in individual experiences are vast. Consider two caregivers losing their spouses – one after a sudden accident, the other after a prolonged illness. The grief experienced will differ profoundly. The sudden loss of the first loss might result in a prolonged period of shock and denial, while the anticipatory grief associated with the long-term illness might lead to a more gradual, albeit equally intense, emotional response. One might express their anger openly, while the other might suppress it, leading to internalized conflict and resentment. Understanding these nuances is crucial for effective support and self-compassion.

Cultural and societal influences also impact how grief is experienced and expressed. Some cultures encourage open displays of emotion, while others emphasize restraint. **Religious beliefs can provide comfort and guidance for some, while others might find solace in secular practices.** These diverse approaches reflect the multitude of ways individuals cope with loss and make sense of their experiences. Recognizing this diversity is vital for respecting the individual's unique grieving journey and providing appropriate support.

Furthermore, external factors like financial strain, family dynamics, and practical challenges significantly impact the grieving process. The added burden of managing finances, navigating bureaucratic processes, and dealing with strained family relationships can exacerbate feelings of exhaustion and overwhelm. These practical realities add further complexity to the already challenging emotional journey. A caregiver might find themselves overwhelmed by paperwork related to estate settlements, while simultaneously grappling with the emotional void left by their loved one's absence. These external pressures often intensify the feelings of helplessness and hopelessness, making it crucial for caregivers to prioritize self-care and seek support networks to manage both the emotional and practical challenges. My two brothers and I had to communicate the best way to make decisions and often it was hard but achievable once a plan was implemented.

Ultimately, the journey through grief is profoundly personal, a uniquely crafted experience shaped by individual circumstances, personality traits, and societal influences. There is no single "right" way to grieve, and there is no timeframe to reach, only navigating the emotions you are feeling. Understanding the varied expressions and intensities of emotions, the non-linear nature of the grieving process, and the unique context of caregiver grief provides a critical foundation for self-compassion, empathy, and effective support.

My intention is to help as many human beings as possible navigate the stages of grief and guide them through the healing process.

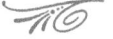

The path forward to your healing journey is not about suppressing or ignoring these emotions, but about acknowledging them, validating them, and finding healthy ways to navigate their intensity. The following chapters will explore specific strategies to support this journey, empowering individuals to find their own path and embrace healing and a renewed sense of well-being and value of who you are now.

Many times during the writing of this book, I faced moments of reality checking and reflection. I saw myself stuck in each one of these stages and realized, "I could have benefited from having my book in hand." My intention for this book is to help as many human beings as possible navigate the stages of grief and guide them through the healing process.

CHAPTER 3

The Physical and Emotional Toll of Grief

The experience of grief, particularly for caregivers, extends far beyond the realm of emotional distress. It deeply impacts physical health, creating a complex interplay between mind and body that can significantly impair well-being. The emotional toll, as we've discussed, is profound and multifaceted, but the physical manifestations are equally significant and often overlooked. Understanding this physical and emotional connection is crucial for effective self-care and navigating the challenging journey of grief.

One of the most common physical symptoms experienced during grief is sleep disturbance. This isn't simply about difficulty falling asleep; it encompasses a range of issues, including insomnia, nightmares, and disrupted sleep cycles. The mind, preoccupied with thoughts of the deceased, struggles to find rest, leaving the body depleted and vulnerable. The constant replay of memories, regrets, or anxieties associated with the loss keeps the caregiver in a state of heightened alertness, preventing the restorative sleep necessary for both physical and emotional recovery. This sleep deprivation, in turn, exacerbates other physical and emotional symptoms, creating a vicious cycle that can be difficult to break.

Studies have shown a strong correlation between sleep disturbances and increased levels of stress hormones, further impacting the body's ability to heal and cope with stress. I struggled with insomnia relying on unhealthy coping mechanisms, such as excessive caffeine or alcohol consumption, which only further disrupted sleep patterns and contributed to my physical health problems over time.

Changes in appetite are another frequently observed physical symptom. Grief can manifest as either increased or decreased appetite, leading to weight loss or gain, both of which pose significant health risks. The loss of appetite can stem from a profound lack of interest in food, a feeling of emptiness that even the most enjoyable meals cannot fill. Conversely, I fluctuated between these extremes, finding comfort in food at times, using it as a coping mechanism to numb emotional pain or deal with feelings of overwhelming sadness. I had moments of both at times I felt completely disconnected from my hunger cues, and other times where food was my only solace.

The emotional toll is profound and multifaceted, but the physical manifestations are equally significant and often overlooked.

This emotional eating, driven by intense feelings, can lead to unhealthy weight gain, increasing the risk of cardiovascular disease, diabetes, and other health complications. The impact on nutritional intake is significant; a caregiver neglecting their dietary needs, whether through lack of interest or overconsumption, weakens their immune system, making them more susceptible to illness and delaying their overall recovery.

Nutritional deficiencies, stemming from either extreme, can exacerbate feelings of fatigue, making it more difficult to cope with the emotional and practical demands of daily life. It was an emotionally driven cycle, difficult to break free from.

Beyond sleep and appetite, grief can manifest as physical pain. This pain is not necessarily linked to a specific injury or illness; instead, it's a psychosomatic response, a manifestation of the emotional distress within the physical body. The symptoms can range from headaches and backaches to chronic pain in various parts of the body. The constant tension and stress associated with grief put a strain on the musculoskeletal system, contributing to muscle aches and joint pain. The physiological changes associated with prolonged stress, such as increased cortisol levels, can also sensitize the body to pain, making even minor discomforts feel more intense.

A caregiver might find themselves experiencing debilitating headaches, migraines, or chronic back pain, significantly impacting their ability to perform daily tasks, both at home and work. It's crucial to acknowledge these physical manifestations of grief and seek appropriate medical attention to address both the physical pain and the underlying emotional distress.

Emotional exhaustion is perhaps the most pervasive and debilitating consequence of prolonged grief, especially for caregivers. The emotional labor involved in providing care, coupled with the emotional turmoil of loss, can lead to complete burnout. This exhaustion is not simply feeling tired; it's a profound depletion of emotional reserves, a state of being where even the simplest tasks feel overwhelming.

Caregivers often report feeling emotionally drained, overwhelmed, and unable to cope with the daily demands of life. This is something I know intimately from my own experience. Juggling a full-time job with the constant demands of caregiving left me feeling perpetually depleted. Evenings, which should have been a time for rest, were often consumed by the additional tasks associated with caregiving, leaving little time for personal needs or simple relaxation. The mental load alone –constantly anticipating needs, problem-solving, and making difficult decisions – was exhausting.

This exhaustion often leaves caregivers vulnerable to other mental health challenges, such as depression and anxiety, compounding the already overwhelming emotional distress. My own experience validated this; the constant pressure led to increased anxiety and periods of profound sadness.

The lack of emotional energy can impact every aspect of a caregiver's life, from their relationships with family and friends to their professional life. I found myself increasingly withdrawn from social activities, unable to muster the energy to engage with friends or even maintain basic communication. At work, my performance suffered, impacting my concentration and ability to meet deadlines. The guilt of not performing adequately in either role added another layer to the already heavy burden.

The inability to adequately care for oneself can lead to neglect of basic self-care routines, further exacerbating both physical and emotional symptoms. This manifested for me in neglecting my diet, exercise, and sleep – a vicious cycle that further depleted my already limited resources. The constant pressure and lack of time and even small acts of self-care, like taking a bath or reading a book, felt impossible to prioritize.

The scientific literature supports the profound impact of grief on physical health. Studies have repeatedly demonstrated a link between prolonged grief and increased risk of cardiovascular disease, respiratory problems, and weakened immune function. For instance, research has shown that individuals experiencing prolonged or complicated grief have a significantly higher risk of developing cardiovascular diseases, such as heart attacks and strokes, compared to their counterparts who have not experienced such profound loss. The constant stress, the sleep disturbances, and the changes in appetite all contribute to the increased risk of cardiovascular complications.

Similarly, studies have explored the impact of grief on the immune system, revealing that prolonged emotional distress can weaken the body's natural defenses, making individuals more susceptible to infections and illnesses. The chronic stress associated with grief can suppress the immune response, leaving the body vulnerable to various health problems. The relationship between emotional distress and respiratory problems is also well-documented, highlighting the interconnectedness between mental and physical health.

Moreover, the experience of anticipatory grief, often experienced by caregivers during a loved one's prolonged illness, adds another layer of complexity to the physical and emotional toll. The prolonged period of emotional preparation for the inevitable loss can be just as emotionally and physically draining as the grief experienced after the death itself. The constant emotional stress, the ongoing worry, and the uncertainty of the future can wear down a caregiver's physical and mental resources, contributing to a state of chronic exhaustion and vulnerability. Anticipatory grief might lead to anticipatory mourning, wherein some of the grieving process begins before the death itself. This can include experiencing some of the physical symptoms mentioned above, such as sleep disturbances, appetite changes, or physical pain, during the period of caregiving before the loss.

It's vital for caregivers to understand this intricate connection between their emotional and physical well-being. Ignoring the physical manifestations of grief only delays healing and can lead to further complications. Seeking support from medical professionals, including doctors and therapists, is crucial for managing both the physical and emotional aspects of grief. This may involve medical intervention to address specific physical symptoms, such as sleep disturbances or chronic pain, alongside therapeutic interventions to address the emotional distress and facilitate the healing process.

Self-care practices, such as mindful exercises, meditation, and engaging in activities that bring joy, become essential tools for managing both the physical and emotional challenges. These practices promote relaxation, reduce stress levels, and help restore a sense of balance and well-being. The journey through grief is long and demanding; prioritizing physical and emotional health is not a luxury, but a necessity for navigating this profound experience with strength and resilience and a path toward healing, fostering a renewed sense of self and a way to honor the memory of the loved one lost.

It is important to keep my loved ones' legacy alive through me loving myself enough to be healthy. This self-care is a tribute to them, a testament to the strength and resilience they instilled in me. By prioritizing my well-being, I am not only honoring their memory but also ensuring their influence continues to shape my life positively.

CHAPTER 4

Recognizing Complicated Grief

G rief is a deeply personal journey, a unique and complex tapestry woven from individual experiences, relationships, and cultural contexts. While the universal experience of loss unites us, the expression and duration of grief vary significantly. Understanding the nuances of this process is crucial, particularly when grief transitions from a natural, albeit painful, response to a more persistent and debilitating condition known as complicated grief. Having watched many loved ones struggle with grief, I've written this book to provide guidance and support. Unlike the natural sadness and adaptation following a loss, complicated grief is a deeply prolonged and overwhelming struggle that severely impacts a person's ability to live their daily life.

My priority is to help those experiencing this intense form of grief navigate it successfully.

Normal grief, while undeniably painful, allows for a gradual process of healing and adaptation. It's characterized by waves of intense emotion, interspersed with moments of relative calm and acceptance. Over time, the intensity of these emotions typically diminishes, allowing the individual to reintegrate into their daily life, build new routines, and find meaning in their experiences. The individual may experience sadness, anger, guilt, or a range of other emotions, but these emotions are manageable and don't completely overwhelm their daily functioning. They can still engage in activities they enjoy, maintain relationships, and attend to personal responsibilities, even if these activities are initially tinged with sadness or require extra effort.

Complicated grief, however, transcends this natural trajectory. It's a condition characterized by persistent and overwhelming distress, significantly interfering with an individual's capacity to cope with daily life. The symptoms are more intense and enduring, often lasting for more than six months, far exceeding the typical grieving period. Instead of a gradual decline in the intensity of emotions, those experiencing complicated grief are often trapped in a cycle of intense sorrow, longing, and disbelief. This prolonged distress can manifest in various ways, impacting all aspects of their lives— emotional, social, physical, and even spiritual. It's crucial to recognize the defining characteristics of complicated grief to distinguish it from the natural process of mourning and to seek timely intervention.

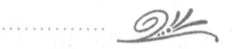

Understanding the nuances of this process is crucial, particularly when grief transitions from a natural, albeit painful, response to a more persistent and debilitating condition known as complicated grief.

One of the key indicators of complicated grief is the persistent and intense yearning for the deceased. This longing isn't simply a wistful remembrance; it's a constant, overwhelming ache, a sense of emptiness that pervades every aspect of their life. Individuals experiencing complicated grief might struggle to accept the reality of the loss, clinging to the hope of reunion or engaging in unrealistic fantasies about the deceased. This disbelief can prevent them from moving forward, creating a sense of being perpetually stuck in the past. It's an emotionally exhausting state, draining their energy and rendering them unable to engage in activities that once brought them joy. The world feels profoundly empty, lacking the vibrant presence of their loved one. Simple tasks, once effortless, can now feel insurmountable, creating a cycle of avoidance and further isolation.

Another significant symptom is the overwhelming sense of numbness or detachment. This isn't just a temporary emotional lull; it's a profound disconnect from life itself. Individuals might feel emotionally paralyzed, unable to experience joy, love, or even basic human connection. The world appears dull, lifeless, and devoid of meaning. This emotional detachment can significantly impact their relationships, making it difficult to engage in meaningful connections with friends, family, or even colleagues. The intensity of this detachment can isolate them further, exacerbating their feelings of loneliness and despair. It can lead to the withdrawal from social interactions, leaving them feeling increasingly isolated and alone in their grief.

The intrusive memories associated with complicated grief are not the gentle reminiscences of normal grief. Instead, they're vivid, intense, and often distressing flashbacks that can be triggered by seemingly innocuous events or objects. These memories are

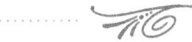

Complicated grief is a deeply prolonged and overwhelming struggle that severely impacts a person's ability to live their daily life.

often accompanied by intense emotional reactions, such as overwhelming sadness, anger, or guilt. These flashbacks are not easily dismissed; they interrupt daily routines, causing significant distress and hindering the ability to concentrate or engage in meaningful activities. The constant recurrence of these vivid memories can overwhelm the individual, making it difficult to focus on anything else. This perpetual revisiting of painful memories prevents the process of healing and acceptance.

Individuals struggling with complicated grief often exhibit significant disruptions in their daily functioning. Simple tasks like getting out of bed, eating, or engaging in self-care can become Herculean efforts.

Their social life often diminishes; participation in previously enjoyed activities diminishes or ceases completely. Their work performance may deteriorate; and relationships with family and friends can suffer, leading to further isolation and compounding their feelings of despair. The intensity of their emotional distress can hinder their ability to maintain their personal hygiene, manage their finances, or even ensure basic physical safety. This significant impairment is a key differentiator from normal grief, highlighting the need for professional intervention.

The intense emotional distress experienced in complicated grief often overlaps with symptoms of other mental health conditions, such as depression and anxiety. Individuals might experience persistent feelings of hopelessness, worthlessness, or an inability to experience pleasure. They might also experience symptoms of anxiety, such as excessive worry, restlessness, and difficulty sleeping. These overlapping conditions further complicate the healing process, requiring a more comprehensive approach to treatment. The presence of depression and anxiety requires a holistic treatment plan addressing both the complicated grief and the co-occurring mental health conditions.

Determining when grief transitions from normal grieving to complicated grief requires careful consideration of the individual's experiences and the persistence of symptoms. While intense emotions are expected after a significant loss, the key differentiators are the duration and the impact on daily functioning. If the intense emotional distress, intrusive memories, and disruptions in daily life persist for more than six months and significantly impair their ability to engage in meaningful activities, professional help should be sought. Ignoring these warning signs can have detrimental consequences, leading to further emotional distress, social isolation, and potential physical health problems.

Professional help can take various forms, depending on the individual's needs and preferences. Therapy, especially cognitive behavioral therapy (CBT) and grief counseling, is particularly beneficial in addressing the cognitive distortions and maladaptive coping mechanisms that often accompany complicated grief.

CBT focuses on identifying and modifying unhelpful thoughts and behaviors, while grief counseling provides a supportive environment to process emotions, explore memories, and develop healthier coping strategies. Medication, such as antidepressants or anti-anxiety medications, might be recommended to address co-occurring mental health conditions, such as depression or anxiety, which frequently accompany complicated grief.

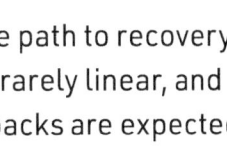

The path to recovery is rarely linear, and setbacks are expected, but with consistent effort and professional support, healing and a renewed sense of purpose are attainable.

Support groups can offer a sense of community and shared understanding, allowing individuals to connect with others who have experienced similar losses. A holistic approach combining therapy, medication, and support groups often yields the best results, supporting a more comprehensive healing process.

Navigating the complexities of grief is a challenging journey.

Seeking professional help isn't a sign of weakness; it's a testament to the individual's courage and commitment to healing. Recognizing the signs of complicated grief and seeking timely intervention is essential for restoring a sense of well-being and reintegrating into life. The healing process requires patience, self-compassion, and a supportive network of professionals and loved ones.

Remember, healing is possible, even from the deepest wounds of grief. The path to recovery is rarely linear, and setbacks are expected, but with consistent effort and professional support, healing and a renewed sense of purpose are attainable. The journey from loss to healing is a journey of profound transformation; and with the right support, it's a journey worth undertaking.

CHAPTER 5

Building a Support System

Building a strong support system is paramount during the grieving process. It's not a sign of weakness to seek help; it's an act of self-preservation and a crucial step to your healing journey. Grief, whether normal or complicated, is a profoundly isolating experience. The intense emotions, the disruption to daily life, and the feeling of being adrift can leave individuals feeling utterly alone, even when surrounded by loved ones. This is where a supportive network becomes not just helpful, but essential.

Your existing relationships can be a cornerstone of your support system. Family members and close friends, if approached with empathy and understanding, can offer invaluable comfort and practical assistance. However, it's important to recognize that not everyone is equipped to provide the level of support you may need. Some friends or family members may struggle to understand the depth of your grief or may inadvertently say or do things that cause further pain. This isn't a reflection on their character, but rather a limitation in their capacity to comprehend the complexities of grief. Their intention may be good, but their actions may not always be helpful I recommended that you guard your heart and follow your inner compass.

Open communication is key. Instead of expecting others to intuit your needs, clearly express what kind of support you require. This could range from practical assistance like meal preparation or childcare to emotional support such as simply listening without judgment. You might need help with errands, transportation, or managing household chores. Let your support network know specifically what would ease your burden. Don't hesitate to state your needs directly, even if it feels awkward. Your friends and family who truly care will want to help, but they might not know how unless you tell them.

For instance, if you find yourself overwhelmed by daily tasks, don't hesitate to ask for help with grocery shopping, cleaning, or running errands. If you're struggling to care for children or pets, openly ask for assistance with their care. If emotional support is what you crave, consider saying something like, "I'm feeling really overwhelmed right now. Could we just sit together and talk, or perhaps just watch a movie together in silence?" Specificity ensures that your support network can provide the assistance you actually need and want, rather than well-meaning but ultimately unhelpful gesture many offer and end up wasting your time.

It's important to remember that your support system may evolve throughout your grieving process. Some people may be able to offer consistent support over the long haul, while others may provide support only during certain phases. This is perfectly acceptable. Grief is a marathon, not a sprint, and your support needs will fluctuate over time. Accepting this ebb and flow is a crucial part of navigating the grieving process.

Beyond family and friends, there are other invaluable sources of support. Support groups offer a unique opportunity to connect with others who are grappling with similar losses. These groups provide a safe space to share experiences, express emotions, and realize you are not alone in your suffering. Hearing others' stories can be incredibly validating and empowering, offering a sense of shared understanding that is often lacking in other social interactions. The shared experience creates a powerful bond that can be incredibly comforting during a difficult time. The opportunity to connect with people who "get it" is invaluable. You'll discover you are not alone in feeling the way you do, and that can ease the burden of isolation.

Support groups are particularly beneficial for those experiencing complicated grief. The sustained intensity of emotions, the pervasive sense of loss, and the difficulty in re-engaging with life can be profoundly isolating. Connecting with others who understand this experience can be immensely comforting.

Remember that there are numerous online support groups offering a geographically diverse and readily accessible community. Online forums allow for more anonymity than face-to-face groups, which can be comforting for individuals who are not yet comfortable sharing their experiences openly.

Professional therapy offers another layer of support. A therapist specializing in grief and loss can provide a safe and confidential space to explore your emotions, identify unhelpful thought patterns, and develop healthier coping mechanisms. They can offer guidance and support as you navigate the complexities of your grief and help you to develop strategies for managing intense emotions and rebuilding your life. A therapist can also help identify any underlying mental health conditions that may be contributing to or exacerbating your grief, ensuring a more comprehensive approach to healing. Therapy is an investment in your long-term well-being, facilitating a more effective and sustainable path towards healing.

Mindfulness and wellness practices, such as meditation, yoga, and spending time in nature, can also be incredibly helpful in managing the emotional intensity of grief. These practices can help to regulate your nervous system, reducing feelings of anxiety and overwhelming sadness. Mindfulness encourages you to focus on the present moment, rather than getting lost in the pain of the past or the anxieties of the future. This focus can offer a sense of calm and stability amidst the turmoil of grief. These practices aren't a cure, but they can provide essential tools for managing emotional distress.

It's crucial to remember that building a support system is an ongoing process. It's not a one-time event; rather, it's a dynamic network that may shift and change over time as your needs evolve.

Be open to seeking support from different sources, and don't be afraid to ask for help. Remember that your healing journey is unique, and finding the right combination of support will likely take time and experimentation.

Consider exploring different approaches, even combining approaches like support groups, therapy, and mindfulness practices.

You might find that certain support methods resonate more with you than others. There's no right or wrong way; what matters is finding what works best for you and makes you feel supported. Be patient with yourself and celebrate small victories along the way.

Healing takes time, and every step you take is building a strong support network that is a step closer to healing. Allow yourself the space and time to explore what works best for your individual needs. Building a strong support system is not merely helpful, it's fundamental to your journey through grief and essential for long-term healing and well-being. It's a continuous process, an evolving network of people and practices that sustain you through the challenges and complexities of loss. Remember, healing is not a linear path, but with commitment and supportive connections, it is certainly possible.

CHAPTER 6

Prioritizing Physical Wellbeing

T he emotional toll of grief can be overwhelming, often overshadowing the importance of physical well-being. However, neglecting your physical health during this already challenging time can significantly hinder your healing process and exacerbate existing difficulties.

Prioritizing your physical health is not a selfish act; it's an important component of self-care and a necessary step for emotional recovery. Think of it as building a strong foundation upon which your emotional healing can reset. A body that's well-nourished, rested, and moving will be better equipped to manage the emotional intensity of the grief that is settling throughout your body.

One of the most fundamental aspects of physical well-being is nutrition. When immersed in grief, it's easy to neglect healthy eating habits.

Think of self-care as building a strong foundation upon which your emotional healing can reset.

The lack of appetite, the emotional exhaustion, and the sheer difficulty of managing daily tasks can lead to poor food choices. However, what we consume directly impacts our energy levels, mood, and overall resilience.

Aim for a balanced diet rich in fruits, vegetables, whole grains, and lean proteins. These foods provide the essential nutrients your body needs to function optimally, particularly during times of stress.

Don't strive for perfection; focus on making small, sustainable changes. Start by incorporating one or two healthy meals into your daily routine. For instance, begin your day with a nutritious breakfast, such as oatmeal with berries and nuts, or a Greek yogurt parfait with fruit and granola. For lunch, opt for a salad with grilled chicken or fish, or a whole-wheat sandwich with plenty of vegetables. Evenings can be simpler; consider light soup or stir-fry with plenty of vegetables and lean protein. Prepare some meals in advance to alleviate the burden of daily cooking and rushed fast food. Consider batch cooking on a weekend to have healthy meals readily available throughout the week these suggestions are those I incorporated on a daily basis.

It's understandable if cooking feels overwhelming. Remember, even small changes matter. Trading processed snacks for fruits and vegetables is a significant step. Adding a serving of vegetables to your dinner or swapping sugary drinks for water can make a difference. If cooking remains a challenge, consider meal delivery services that offer healthy options, or enlist the help of friends or family for meal preparation. Reaching out for support is not a sign of weakness; it's a strategic way to prioritize your health.

Beyond nutrition, regular physical activity is crucial for both physical and mental health. Exercise releases endorphins, natural mood boosters that can help combat feelings of sadness and anxiety. It also helps to regulate sleep patterns and reduce stress levels—all essential during grief. However, it's important to approach exercise realistically. You don't need to engage in strenuous workouts; even moderate activity can make a significant difference.

Start with short, manageable walks. A 15-20 minute walk daily can significantly improve your mood and energy levels. If walking is difficult, try gentle stretches or chair exercises. There are numerous online resources offering simple chair exercises suitable for all fitness levels. As your stamina increases, gradually increase the duration and intensity of your workouts. Remember to listen to your body and rest when needed. The goal is to find an activity that you enjoy and that fits seamlessly into your daily routine.

Sleep is another vital component of physical well-being. Grief can significantly disrupt sleep patterns, leading to insomnia, fatigue, and reduced cognitive function. Aim for 7-8 hours of quality sleep each night. Establish a regular sleep schedule, even on weekends.

Create a relaxing bedtime routine to signal to your body that it's time to rest. This could include a warm bath, reading a book, or listening to calming music. Minimize screen time before bed, as the blue light emitted from electronic devices can interfere with sleep. If you're struggling with insomnia, consider consulting your doctor or a sleep specialist.

Stress management is equally important. Grief is inherently stressful, and chronic stress can have detrimental effects on both physical and mental health. Explore various stress-reduction techniques and find what works best for you. Deep breathing exercises can help to calm your nervous system and reduce feelings of anxiety. Progressive muscle relaxation, a technique that involves tensing and releasing different muscle groups, can help to alleviate physical tension associated with stress. Mindfulness meditation, as discussed previously, can also be incredibly beneficial in managing stress and fostering a sense of calm.

> Reaching out for support is not a sign of weakness; it's a strategic way to prioritize your health.

Consider incorporating enjoyable activities into your daily routine to counteract the stress of grief. This could include spending time in nature, listening to music, reading, engaging in a hobby, or spending time with loved ones. These activities provide a welcome distraction and offer a sense of normalcy during a challenging time. Remember that self-care is not a luxury; it's a necessity, especially during times of grief. Prioritizing your physical well-being is an act of self-compassion and a critical step for healing.

Consider the practicality of incorporating these self-care practices into the life of a caregiver. Time is often limited, and exhaustion is common. Simple, manageable exercises are crucial. Five minutes of stretching each morning, followed by a short walk during a break in the day, can make a big difference. Similarly, focus on quick, healthy meals that require minimal preparation. Pre-cut vegetables, canned beans, and whole-grain bread can be combined quickly for a nutritious meal. Utilize a slow cooker or Instant Pot to prepare meals in advance. Remember, a perfectly healthy diet isn't necessary; small, incremental changes in food choices are a massive step for improved wellbeing. Instead of feeling the pressure of a complete lifestyle overhaul, focus on achievable steps that will maintain consistency over time.

If you're struggling to fit in self-care, create a realistic schedule. This schedule could include specific times for exercise, healthy meals, and periods of relaxation. Even small pockets of time, like 10-15 minutes throughout the day, can be dedicated to deep breathing or meditation. Treat these scheduled self-care activities as non-negotiable appointments; don't allow them to be displaced by other tasks. Remember, taking care of yourself is not selfish but essential for your ability to care for others. If you're finding it challenging to prioritize self-care independently, ask a trusted friend or family member for assistance.

In the whirlwind of grief and caregiving responsibilities, it's easy to put your needs last. However, your ability to offer effective care to others is deeply connected to your own well-being. Remember, a caregiver who is physically and emotionally exhausted is less able to cope with the demands of caregiving. By prioritizing your physical health, you are not only improving your own well-being but also strengthening your capacity to provide care for others.

It's a virtuous cycle: taking care of yourself empowers you to take better care of others, and supporting others creates a sense of purpose and can contribute to your own healing. Consider self-care as an investment in your long-term health, both emotional and physical. It's not a luxury, but a vital strategy for navigating the complexities of grief and caregiving. Remember to be patient with yourself; progress is made one small step at a time.

CHAPTER 7

Mindfulness and Meditation for Grief

Mindfulness and meditation offer powerful tools for navigating the turbulent waters of grief. These practices, rooted in present-moment awareness, can help caregivers cultivate emotional regulation, reduce stress, and foster a sense of inner peace amidst the challenges of loss and caregiving responsibilities. Unlike other coping mechanisms that might offer temporary relief, mindfulness and meditation provide a sustainable approach to managing the emotional intensity associated with grief, allowing for a deeper connection to one's inner strength and resilience.

> Mindfulness is about acknowledging and accepting all thoughts and feelings without getting carried away by them.

These practices, rooted in present-moment awareness, can help caregivers cultivate emotional regulation, reduce stress, and foster a sense of inner peace amidst the challenges of loss and caregiving responsibilities. Unlike other coping mechanisms that might offer temporary relief, mindfulness and meditation provide a sustainable approach to managing the emotional intensity associated with grief, allowing for a deeper connection to one's inner strength and resilience.

The core principle of mindfulness lies in paying attention to the present moment without judgment. This seemingly simple act can be profoundly transformative when facing grief. Instead of getting caught in the cycle of ruminating on the past or anxiously anticipating the future, mindfulness encourages a gentle return to the here and now. This shift in focus can interrupt the overwhelming emotions often associated with grief, providing a space for calmer reflection and emotional processing.

A common misconception is that mindfulness requires emptying the mind. This is not the case. Mindfulness is about acknowledging and accepting all thoughts and feelings without getting carried away by them. Thoughts and emotions, even painful ones, are simply fleeting experiences, like clouds passing across the sky. The practice is about observing these internal states without becoming entangled in their intensity. It's about creating a space for emotional awareness without judgment, allowing grief to be experienced without resistance.

Several techniques can cultivate mindfulness. One simple method is focusing on the breath. Find a comfortable position, either sitting or lying down, and gently bring your attention to the sensation of your breath as it enters and leaves your body. Notice the rise and fall of your chest or abdomen. When your mind wanders—and it inevitably will—gently redirect your attention back to your breath. Don't criticize yourself for getting distracted; simply acknowledge the distraction and return to your breath. This exercise, even practiced for just five minutes a day, can significantly enhance your ability to stay grounded in the present.

Another helpful technique is body scan meditation. This involves systematically bringing awareness to different parts of your body, noticing any sensations without judgment. Start with your toes, paying attention to any tingling, warmth, or tension. Slowly move your awareness up your body, noticing sensations in your feet, ankles, calves, and so on. This practice cultivates body awareness, which can be particularly helpful in managing the physical manifestations of stress and grief, such as muscle tension or digestive discomfort.

Mindfulness can be incorporated into daily activities, transforming ordinary tasks into opportunities for present-moment awareness. While washing dishes, for instance, focus on the warmth of the water, the feel of the soap, and the sound of the water running. While walking, notice the texture of the pavement under your feet, the sights and sounds around you, and the rhythm of your steps.

This approach helps to cultivate a sense of presence and appreciation for the simple things in life, counteracting the pervasive negativity that grief can bring.

Meditation, a more formal practice of mindfulness, involves focusing on a specific object, such as the breath, a mantra, or a visual image. Meditation helps to quiet the mind and cultivate a sense of inner peace. Guided meditations are particularly beneficial for those new to the practice, providing a structured approach and verbal cues to guide your attention. Numerous guided meditations for grief are available online or through meditation apps.

The benefits of meditation for grief extend beyond simply calming the mind. Regular meditation practice can help to reduce stress hormones, improve sleep quality, boost the immune system, and enhance emotional regulation. It can also promote self-compassion, a crucial component of healing from grief. By cultivating self-compassion, you learn to treat yourself with the same kindness and understanding that you would offer a close friend facing a similar loss.

When beginning a meditation practice, start with short sessions (5-10 minutes) and gradually increase the duration as you become more comfortable. Consistency is key. Even short, regular sessions can provide significant benefits. Find a quiet space where you won't be disturbed, and make sure you're comfortable. You can meditate sitting on a cushion, lying down, or even sitting in a chair. Experiment with different positions to find what works best for you.

It's essential to approach mindfulness and meditation with patience and self-compassion. Don't get discouraged if your mind wanders or you find it difficult to focus. These are normal experiences. Simply acknowledge the distractions and gently redirect your attention back to your chosen focus. Remember, the goal is not to achieve a state of perfect stillness but to cultivate a greater awareness of your thoughts, feelings, and bodily sensations.

Many guided meditation scripts are specifically designed to support individuals experiencing grief. These scripts often include gentle prompts to acknowledge feelings, release tension, and cultivate self-compassion. For example, a guided meditation might begin by inviting you to focus on your breath, then gently guide you through a body scan, noticing any areas of tension or discomfort. The script might then offer supportive affirmations or visualizations to help you connect with your inner strength and resilience.

Taking care of yourself is not selfish; it's essential for your continued ability to care for others.

The integration of mindfulness and meditation into daily life can be a transformative experience for caregivers grappling with grief. By incorporating these practices into your routine, you cultivate a greater capacity for self-awareness, emotional regulation, and stress management. This, in turn, enhances your ability to provide compassionate care to others while nurturing your own well-being.

This is not merely a form of self-care; it's a fundamental component of sustainable caregiving, ensuring that your capacity for compassion isn't depleted, enabling you to navigate the complexities of grief and caregiving with greater resilience and inner peace. Remember, taking care of yourself is not selfish; it's essential for your continued ability to care for others. The journey of grief is long and complex, and these practices can offer a lifeline of support and guidance along the way. Consistency and patience are key; the benefits will unfold gradually, enriching your ability to both grieve and care with greater self-awareness and emotional well-being.

CHAPTER 8

The Power of Journaling and Creative Expression

The profound emotional landscape of grief often leaves individuals feeling overwhelmed and unable to articulate the hard to handle tapestry of feelings they experience. While mindfulness and meditation offer invaluable tools for cultivating inner peace and emotional regulation, the act of expressing these emotions through journaling and other creative outlets can be equally transformative.

Journaling, in particular, provides a safe and private space to explore the depths of grief without judgment, allowing for a deeper understanding of the emotional process. It's a powerful tool for processing the myriad of emotions – sadness, anger, guilt, confusion, and even moments of peace – that often accompany loss.

> The simple act of putting pen to paper can unlock a release of pent-up emotions that may otherwise remain trapped within.

The simple act of putting pen to paper, or fingers to keyboard, can unlock a release of pent-up emotions that may otherwise remain trapped within. It's not about creating a polished piece of prose; it's about allowing the raw, unfiltered emotions to flow freely onto the page. This process can be surprisingly cathartic, providing a sense of emotional release and validation. The journal becomes a witness to your grief, a silent confidante in the journey of healing.

Consider these journaling prompts as starting points to guide your exploration:

"Describe a vivid memory of the person you lost." This prompt encourages you to engage with positive memories, fostering a sense of connection and remembering the essence of the departed. Allow yourself to delve into the sensory details: what did they smell like? What was the sound of their laughter? What emotions did you associate with them?

"Write a letter to the person you lost." This can be a profoundly healing exercise. Pour out your heart, expressing your unexpressed feelings, unresolved issues, and lingering questions. There is no need for censorship; allow yourself to be completely honest and vulnerable.

"What are three words that describe your feelings today?" This exercise helps you to identify and label your emotions in the present moment, a crucial step in processing them. It fosters self-awareness and offers a concise way to track the ebb and flow of your emotional state.

"What are three things you are grateful for today?" While seemingly at odds with the profound sadness of grief, practicing gratitude can help shift your perspective, even slight moments of appreciation and positivity, offering a counterbalance to the dominant feelings of loss.

"Describe a recent dream you've had." Dreams often reflect the subconscious processing of emotions and experiences. Reflecting on your dreams can offer valuable insights into how your subconscious mind is grappling with your grief.

Beyond journaling, numerous other creative outlets can serve as powerful tools for emotional expression and processing. Art therapy, for instance, allows individuals to externalize their inner turmoil through visual representations. The act of painting, sculpting, drawing, or engaging in other visual arts can be a cathartic experience, allowing for a non-verbal expression of emotions too complex to articulate verbally. The colors, shapes, and textures chosen can reveal deeper aspects of one's emotional landscape.

Music therapy offers another avenue for emotional expression. Playing a musical instrument, singing, or simply listening to music can evoke powerful emotions and memories. The rhythm, melody, and lyrics can resonate with your emotional state, providing a sense of solace and connection. Experimenting with different genres and styles can help you explore the vast spectrum of your emotions.

Similarly, writing poetry, fiction, or even simply free writing can offer a creative means of processing grief. The act of crafting words, images, and metaphors can facilitate a deeper understanding of your emotional experience, enabling you to transform raw pain into something beautiful and meaningful. Don't worry about adhering to strict literary rules or technical perfection; the primary goal is to create an outlet for your emotions.

It's important to emphasize that there's no "right" or "wrong" way to engage in these creative processes. The goal is not to produce a masterpiece but to utilize these outlets as tools for self-discovery and emotional regulation. Allow yourself to explore different mediums, experiment with different approaches, and discover which resonates most deeply with your individual needs. Be patient and compassionate with yourself; the process may be challenging at times, but it can ultimately be transformative.

Moreover, the creative process doesn't have to be solitary. Sharing your creative work with a trusted friend, family member, or therapist can provide a sense of connection and validation. It can also provide an opportunity to receive support and understanding from others. However, remember that this is entirely optional; the primary benefit of these activities comes from the personal act of self-expression.

The act of creatively expressing your grief doesn't necessarily alleviate the pain entirely; instead, it transforms the relationship with it. It's about finding a constructive means of engaging with your grief, turning a chaotic torrent of emotions into a more manageable stream. This process of creating order from chaos isn't about erasing the pain but about creating a new relationship with it – one that fosters understanding, acceptance, and eventually, healing. This creative engagement helps to move beyond simply enduring grief to actively shaping one's experience of it. It's about claiming your story, not necessarily to rewrite it, but to understand it better, and to find strength and meaning within its complexities.

> This creative engagement helps to move beyond simply enduring grief to actively shaping one's experience of it.

Remember, the process of grieving is not linear; there will be days when the creative well feels dry, where the emotions feel too overwhelming to articulate. On such days, it's perfectly acceptable to simply allow yourself to rest and be present in your grief, without pressure to force creative expression. The key is to establish a regular practice – even brief sessions of journaling or sketching – that cultivates a consistent space for self-expression. Just as mindfulness and meditation provide regular check-ins with your inner state, creative expression offers a means of communicating that inner world to yourself and, if you choose, to others.

Over time, this consistent engagement with your emotional world through creative outlets fosters a deeper sense of self-awareness. You begin to recognize patterns in your emotional responses, understand the triggers that evoke specific feelings, and identify healthier ways to manage your grief. This self-awareness is crucial for building resilience and developing coping mechanisms that will serve you long after the acute phase of grief has subsided. The creative process becomes, in essence, a tool for ongoing self-discovery, empowering you to navigate the complexities of loss with greater clarity, self-compassion, and strength.

Furthermore, the integration of journaling and creative expression into your self-care routine is not just about healing from the past; it also plays a vital role in building a stronger, more resilient future.

By consistently expressing your emotions, you create a record of your journey, a testament to your inner strength and resilience. This record can serve as a source of comfort and inspiration during challenging times, reminding you of your capacity to navigate difficult emotions and emerge stronger on the other side. It's a reminder that you are not defined by your grief, but by your ability to find meaning and purpose amidst loss. It's about finding beauty in the brokenness, strength in vulnerability, and hope in the midst of despair.

Your story is unique, and your journey of grief is your own; these creative tools offer a path towards understanding, acceptance, and healing. Embrace the process, however messy or uncomfortable it may be, and allow yourself the time and space to navigate the complexities of your grief with compassion and grace.

CHAPTER 9

Setting Healthy Boundaries

T he emotional toll of caregiving, especially when compounded by grief, can be immense. It's easy to become overwhelmed, to prioritize the needs of others above your own until you're left depleted and unable to effectively support anyone, including yourself. Setting healthy boundaries isn't selfish; it's essential for your well-being and your ability to continue providing care. It's about recognizing your limits and communicating them clearly and respectfully to others.

> This is about sustaining your capacity to provide effective compassionate care, healthy over the long haul.

Think of your energy as a finite resource. Just as you wouldn't expect your car to run indefinitely without refueling, you cannot endlessly pour yourself into caregiving without replenishing your own reserves. Setting boundaries is like managing your fuel gauge: you're actively monitoring your energy levels and taking steps to prevent running on empty. This isn't about withdrawing from those you care for; it's about sustaining your capacity to provide effective and compassionate care, healthy over the long haul.

One of the most challenging, yet crucial, aspects of setting healthy boundaries is learning to say "no." This might involve declining extra responsibilities, turning down social invitations when you need time to rest, or politely refusing requests that strain your already limited resources. **This can feel counterintuitive, especially if you're accustomed to putting others' needs first.** However, saying "no" protects your energy, preventing burnout and allowing you to focus your attention where it's most needed.

Consider this scenario: you're caring for an aging parent, juggling work commitments, and managing your own household. A friend calls asking you to help them move furniture that weekend. While you'd love to help, you know that adding this task to your plate would leave you completely exhausted and potentially jeopardize your ability to care for your parent. Learning to politely decline –"Thank you for thinking of me, but I'm completely booked this weekend. I hope you find someone to help you!" – preserves your energy and protects your well-being.

The key to saying "no" effectively lies in the way you communicate it. Avoid guilt or excessive explanation. A simple and direct "no" is often sufficient. If you feel the need to offer an explanation, keep it brief and focus on your existing commitments. For example, instead of saying, "I'm so sorry, I can't help you move because I'm already overwhelmed and I'm really struggling to keep up with everything," try, "Thank you for asking, but I won't be available this weekend." This avoids getting bogged down in justifications and minimizes the chance of feeling pressured to change your mind.

Delegating tasks is another vital aspect of boundary setting. This doesn't necessarily mean relinquishing control; rather, it's about recognizing that you don't have to do everything yourself. Perhaps a family member can assist with meal preparation, errands, or household chores. If you're struggling financially, exploring community resources or hiring help (even for a few hours a week) can provide invaluable support. This doesn't signify failure; it's a strategic allocation of tasks to maximize efficiency and minimize your burden.

Imagine you're responsible for all aspects of your loved one's medical appointments, medication management, and personal care. This is an enormous undertaking, and it's likely to lead to burnout. Could a sibling or other family member help with scheduling appointments or running errands? Could you hire a home health aide to assist with personal care for a few hours each week? These seemingly small delegations can dramatically reduce your workload and prevent emotional exhaustion.

The art of delegation requires clear communication and a willingness to trust others. Begin by identifying tasks that can be shared. Then, approach potential helpers with a specific request, explaining the importance of their assistance and the impact it would have on your well-being. For instance, you could say, "I'm feeling overwhelmed trying to manage everything related to Dad's appointments. Would you be willing to help me schedule his next doctor's visit?" This direct and collaborative approach facilitates a shared responsibility, alleviating some of the pressure you're experiencing.

Beyond family and friends, explore community resources that can provide support. Senior centers, churches, community organizations, and home health agencies often offer services such as meal delivery, transportation, companionship, and respite care. These resources can significantly reduce your workload and provide much-needed time for self-care. Don't hesitate to seek assistance –it's a sign of strength, not weakness.

Seeking professional help is not a sign of failure but a demonstration of self-awareness and commitment to your well-being. Therapists specializing in grief and loss can provide invaluable support, helping you navigate your emotions, develop coping mechanisms, and build resilience. Support groups offer a safe and supportive environment to connect with others who understand your experience. Consider these options not as a last resort, but as essential tools to help you maintain your physical and emotional health during a challenging time. Remember, you cannot pour from an empty cup. Prioritizing your well-being is not selfish; it's essential for your ability to care for others.

Role-playing can be a useful tool for practicing boundary setting. Imagine a scenario where someone is making unreasonable demands on your time or energy. Practice responding assertively but kindly. For example, if someone persistently calls you at inconvenient times, you can practice saying, "I'm happy to talk, but it's difficult for me to answer the phone after 8 pm. Would you mind calling me earlier tomorrow?" Rehearsing these responses can boost your confidence and make it easier to set boundaries in real-life situations.

Consider a scenario where a well-meaning friend keeps offering unsolicited advice. Practice responding by saying something like, "I appreciate your concern, but I'm handling things in my own way right now." Or, if someone is consistently overstepping boundaries in your home, you can practice a clear and direct statement such as, "I need some personal space right now. Could you please give me some time alone?" These scenarios help you anticipate challenging situations and develop effective communication strategies.

Remember that setting boundaries is an ongoing process. It requires consistent practice, patience, and self-compassion. There will be times when you falter, when you say "yes" when you should have said "no." This is perfectly normal. The key is to learn from these experiences and to continue striving to protect your well-being. Don't be afraid to readjust your boundaries as needed; your needs may change over time, and your boundaries should reflect those changes.

Prioritize self-care activities that help you replenish your energy and manage stress. This might involve exercise, meditation, spending time in nature, engaging in hobbies, or connecting with supportive friends and family. These activities are not luxuries; they are essential for maintaining your overall well-being.

By integrating self-care practices into your routine, you're not merely tending to your own needs; you're forging the robust foundation essential for navigating the profound demands of caregiving and the intricate journey of grief. Remember, nurturing your own well-being is never a selfish act; it is, in fact, the most crucial component of providing effective, compassionate, and sustainable care for others. Your capacity to extend support is directly proportional to the strength of your own reserves, and establishing healthy boundaries is the indispensable key to unlocking and preserving that vital capacity.

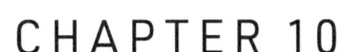

CHAPTER 10

Managing Guilt and Self Blame

The relentless demands of caregiving, especially when intertwined with the profound sorrow of loss, can often create a challenging landscape where feelings of guilt and self-blame take root. This is a common, yet often isolating, experience. The constant worry about whether you are doing "enough," combined with emotional exhaustion, can lead to a persistent internal dialogue filled with self-criticism and regret. You might find yourself questioning past decisions, replaying difficult moments, and agonizing over perceived shortcomings. This inner critic, whispering doubts and accusations, can become a significant barrier to your own well-being and your capacity to continue providing compassionate care.

Understanding that these feelings are a natural part of the human experience is the first crucial step toward easing their burden. Grief itself often involves a complex tapestry of emotions, including regret, remorse, and a profound sense of responsibility. When these are combined with the immense pressures of caregiving, such feelings can be amplified, creating an overwhelming sense of guilt. It's easy to find yourself blaming yourself for circumstances beyond your control, for things you could not have prevented, or for the simple, painful reality that loss is an unavoidable aspect of life.

This self-blame can manifest in various ways. You might criticize your past actions, wishing you had made different choices or handled situations differently. Perhaps you feel a sense of inadequacy in your caregiving role, comparing yourself to others whom you perceive as managing effortlessly. This constant comparison and self-criticism can lead to feelings of worthlessness and despair. It is vital to remember that caregiving is not a competition, and there is no single "right" way to provide care. What truly matters is your dedication, your compassion, and the genuine love you offer.

> Understanding that these feelings are a natural part of the human experience is the first crucial step toward easing the burden.

The key to navigating this guilt and self-blame lies in gently challenging the negative self-talk that fuels it. This involves cultivating self-compassion, actively questioning unhelpful thoughts, and reframing your perception of the situation. Self-compassion is the practice of treating yourself with the same kindness, understanding, and patience you would offer a dear friend facing similar struggles. It's about recognizing that you are human, that mistakes are an inevitable part of any complex journey, and that your inherent worth is not determined by your ability to flawlessly navigate the complexities of caregiving and grief.

One effective technique is **cognitive restructuring**, a process of identifying and challenging negative thought patterns. When you find yourself caught in a cycle of self-criticism, pause and ask yourself: *Is this thought truly accurate? Is there another, more compassionate way to interpret this situation? What advice would I offer a friend facing this same challenge?* By questioning the validity of your negative thoughts and actively seeking alternative, more balanced perspectives, you can begin to dismantle the foundations of self-blame.

Let's consider some examples. Imagine you are caring for a parent with dementia. You might find yourself thinking, "I should have noticed the signs sooner," or "I'm a terrible child for not being able to prevent this." These are common, painful thoughts, often fueled by grief and a deep sense of responsibility. However, through cognitive restructuring, you can gently challenge them. You might reframe the thought: "While I wish I had recognized the signs earlier, it's impossible to know exactly when the disease began. Blaming myself doesn't change what happened. I am doing my very best now, and that is what truly matters." Or "My love and dedication haven't diminished simply because this disease has progressed. Being a 'good' child means offering love and support through difficult times, not preventing illness."

Writing out specific situations where you feel guilt, followed by your challenging thoughts and alternative perspectives, can help solidify your cognitive restructuring practices, creating a tangible record of your progress in managing self-blame.

Finally, remember that seeking professional support is a profound sign of strength, not weakness.

Therapy can provide valuable tools for challenging negative thoughts, managing overwhelming emotions, and developing healthier self-care habits. Group therapy, specifically those tailored to caregivers, can also provide a powerful sense of community and shared experience.

Self-forgiveness is a critical aspect of healing. It's not about condoning your actions; it's about recognizing your humanity, accepting your imperfections, and learning from your experiences. It's about understanding that you did the best you could with the resources you had at the time. It involves recognizing that while you may have made mistakes, you are not defined by them. It's a process that unfolds gradually, requiring patience, self-compassion, and the willingness to let go of the burden of self-blame.

Actively engaging in self-care activities becomes vital in managing these overwhelming emotions. Prioritizing self-care is not selfish; it's a fundamental necessity for your ability to continue providing care effectively and compassionately. Identify activities that bring you joy, relaxation, and a sense of rejuvenation. These could include anything from spending time in nature, pursuing hobbies, reading, listening to music, engaging in gentle exercise, or connecting with supportive friends and family. These activities help replenish your emotional reserves and provide a much-needed break from the intensity of caregiving. Regular, even small, acts of self-care can have a significant impact on your well-being and your resilience.

The experience of guilt and self-blame among caregivers is prevalent and understandable given the complex emotional landscape they navigate. However, by learning to challenge negative self-talk, practice self-compassion, utilize cognitive restructuring techniques, and engage in mindfulness and self-care, you can gradually reclaim your emotional well-being.

Remember that professional support is a vital resource, offering guidance and support as you navigate these challenges. The journey toward self-forgiveness and emotional healing is a personal one, requiring time, patience, and self-compassion. But with consistent effort and the right tools, you can emerge stronger, more resilient, and better equipped to manage the demands of caregiving while prioritizing your own well-being.

CHAPTER 11

Understanding and Processing Anger

nger, a potent and often overwhelming emotion, frequently emerges in the wake of loss. It's a natural response to the disruption, injustice, and pain that grief inflicts. While sadness and guilt may be more readily associated with bereavement, anger often simmers beneath the surface, sometimes erupting unexpectedly, other times manifesting as a low-grade simmering resentment. Understanding this anger, its origins, and its impact is crucial to navigating the complex emotional landscape of grief.

The anger you experience may be directed at different targets. It might be aimed at the deceased: a feeling of betrayal or abandonment for leaving you behind. This is particularly common when the loss was sudden or unexpected, leaving unresolved issues and unmet needs. The intensity of this anger can be amplified if there were unresolved conflicts or unspoken words before the death. You might find yourself replaying arguments or wishing you had said something different, leading to profound regret and anger at the unchangeable past. This is a normal response, though it can be incredibly painful. Allowing yourself to acknowledge and feel this anger without judgment is an essential part of processing it.

Alternatively, anger might be directed at yourself. This self-directed anger often stems from feelings of guilt, regret, or inadequacy related to the circumstances of the loss. You might berate yourself for perceived failures, missed opportunities, or things you wish you had done differently. This self-criticism can be especially harsh and debilitating. The key here is to recognize that this self-directed anger is often a manifestation of grief itself, not an accurate reflection of your worth or value.

Understanding and processing anger while navigating grief is a complex, yet essential, aspect of healing. This powerful emotion can be directed towards various individuals or circumstances, including family members, friends, healthcare professionals, or even broader institutions. For instance, if a loved one's death resulted from negligence or a preventable accident, anger directed at those perceived as responsible is a natural and often justifiable response. It is important to acknowledge the validity of these feelings and allow yourself to express them in healthy, constructive ways. However, it is equally crucial to ensure this anger does not consume you or inadvertently damage the very relationships that offer vital support during this challenging time.

Furthermore, anger can manifest as profound frustration with the perceived unfairness of life, the randomness of loss, and the seemingly arbitrary nature of death. This "existential anger" can be particularly challenging to address, as it confronts the very foundations of our belief systems. It can feel like a deep sense of injustice, a rebellion against the natural order of things. This type of anger often requires deep introspection and potentially a reassessment of your beliefs about the world and your place within it. Exploring your spiritual or philosophical perspectives, or engaging in contemplative practices such as meditation or journaling, can be helpful avenues for processing these complex emotions.

Effectively managing anger is paramount to your emotional and physical well-being during this difficult period. Suppressing your anger is rarely a productive strategy; it often leads to resentment, can manifest as physical symptoms, and may even intensify the anger later on. Instead, finding healthy outlets for expressing your anger is crucial.

Physical activity, for instance, can be a powerful tool for releasing pent-up energy and emotion. Other strategies include talking openly with a trusted friend or therapist, engaging in creative expression, or utilizing mindfulness practices to observe and acknowledge the anger without judgment, allowing it to dissipate naturally with managing intense emotions. A vigorous workout, a brisk walk, or even a focused yoga session can help release pent-up energy and provide a healthy channel for expressing anger. The physical release of endorphins can also have a calming effect.

Assertive communication is another effective strategy. This doesn't mean being aggressive or confrontational; rather, it's about expressing your feelings clearly and respectfully, while still setting boundaries. If you feel anger toward a specific individual, practice expressing your anger directly but calmly. Use "I" statements, focusing on how you feel rather than placing blame. For example, instead of saying, "You made me so angry," try "I felt angry and hurt when..." This approach minimizes defensiveness and promotes a more productive conversation.

Examples of assertive communication. Imagine you're angry with a family member who made insensitive comments about your grief. Instead of lashing out, you could say, "I understand you may not have intended to hurt me, but your comments about [the deceased's name] being 'better off' were deeply upsetting. I need some space to process my grief without feeling judged." This conveys your feelings directly and respectfully, while setting a clear boundary.

Another scenario: You're angry with a healthcare professional who you feel wasn't attentive to your loved one's needs. You could calmly and directly express your concern: "I felt frustrated and angry that my concerns about [specific concern] were not adequately addressed. I'm hoping we can work together to improve communication and ensure that future patients receive better care." Again, this assertive approach avoids blame while communicating your feelings and expectations clearly.

Remember that anger doesn't always need to be overtly expressed. Sometimes, simply acknowledging its presence and allowing yourself to feel it is sufficient. This can be done through journaling where you write about the specifics of what triggered your anger and how it felt in your body. This act of acknowledging and processing your feelings can significantly lessen its intensity over time.

Creative outlets can also be beneficial. Engaging in activities like painting, writing poetry, playing music, or sculpting can allow you to express your anger indirectly, channeling it into a creative expression. This method provides a healthy outlet without requiring direct confrontation or verbal expression. These outlets can be particularly effective in processing complex or deeply rooted anger related to existential issues.

Additionally, support groups can provide invaluable support. Sharing your anger with others who understand the experience of grief can lessen feelings of isolation and provide a sense of validation. Hearing other people's stories and learning how they manage their anger can be incredibly helpful and empowering. Knowing you are not alone in your experience can be a source of strength and resilience.

Remember that seeking professional help is a sign of strength, not weakness. A therapist can provide a safe space to explore your anger, understand its root causes, and develop healthy coping mechanisms. They can guide you through challenging situations and equip you with the skills needed to navigate your grief effectively. Therapy offers a structured environment for processing complex emotions and establishing healthy behavioral patterns.

Remember, anger is a normal and often powerful response to loss. While navigating anger requires patience and self-awareness, actively employing healthy coping mechanisms can profoundly enhance your emotional well-being throughout the grieving process. These include engaging in physical activity, practicing assertive communication, expressing yourself through journaling, exploring creative outlets, and seeking professional support. Allowing yourself to experience and process your anger, rather than suppressing it, is a critical step toward genuine healing and discovering a path forward.

CHAPTER 12

Coping With Guilt and Regret

G uilt and regret are insidious companions to grief, often lurking beneath the surface of more readily apparent emotions like anger and sadness. These feelings can be particularly pervasive for caregivers, who may grapple with the belief that they could have done something differently to prevent the loss or alleviate the suffering of their loved one. This self-blame, while deeply painful, is a common and understandable response to the complexities of death and dying. It's crucial to understand that these feelings are not necessarily indicative of personal failings, but rather a manifestation of the intense emotional upheaval associated with loss.

The first step in coping with guilt and regret is acknowledging their presence. Suppressing these feelings will only amplify their power, causing them to fester and potentially disrupt your emotional well-being.

Allow yourself to feel the weight of these emotions without judgment. Create a safe space, perhaps through journaling, meditation, or simply spending time in nature, where you can explore these feelings without the pressure of immediate resolution.

Recognize that these emotions are part of the grieving process, a testament to the depth of your love and connection with the loss of your loved one.

Cognitive behavioral therapy (CBT) offers valuable tools for challenging negative thought patterns associated with guilt and regret. CBT focuses on identifying and altering unhelpful thought processes, replacing them with more realistic and balanced perspectives. When confronted with feelings of guilt, ask yourself: "What evidence supports this thought?" Often, the reality is far more nuanced than the initial negative assessment. For example, if you're burdened by the belief that you didn't spend enough time with your loved one, consider the totality of your relationship. Remember the cherished moments, the shared laughter, the unconditional love. Acknowledge the limitations of time and circumstances.

It's rare that anyone feels they spent enough time with a loved one after they're gone. This feeling of inadequacy, of wishing you'd had the resources or guidance to navigate your grief more effectively, is common. I, myself, realized I was stuck in a kind of numb despair, regretting the lost opportunity to process my grief in a healthier way. Having the right tools – a framework for understanding the stages of grief, coping mechanisms, and support systems – would have made a profound difference. That's why understanding and utilizing these resources is so crucial. They can help prevent the sense of helplessness and wasted time that can accompany grief.

Replacing self-criticism with self-compassion is another vital element of CBT in the context of grief. Self-compassion involves treating yourself with the same kindness, understanding, and acceptance you would offer a close friend facing a similar loss. Imagine your best friend experiencing the same overwhelming guilt; what would you say to them? Would you berate them for their perceived failings, or would you offer solace, support, and reassurance? Extend that same compassion to yourself.

Acknowledge your own struggles and vulnerabilities without resorting to self-recrimination. Consider the specific situations fueling your guilt or regret. Were there unresolved conflicts? Unspoken words? Missed opportunities? Reflect on these scenarios objectively, acknowledging the complexity of human relationships and the limitations of human capabilities. Perfection is unattainable; we all make mistakes and have regrets. The absence of perfection doesn't equate to failure or worthlessness. Understanding this fundamental truth can significantly reduce the burden of self-blame.

Let's explore some examples of how to apply CBT techniques in the context of caregiver guilt. Imagine you are stuck with the guilt of not recognizing the early signs of your loved one's illness. The negative thought might be: "If I had only been more observant, I could have intervened sooner, and they wouldn't have suffered so much." This is a common and understandable feeling, but it's crucial to challenge its validity. **Ask yourself**: "What evidence supports the belief that I could have definitively recognized the early signs?" Often, early symptoms are subtle and ambiguous, making early detection incredibly difficult. Medical diagnoses can be challenging, and even with expert medical advice, outcomes can be unpredictable. Instead of dwelling on what you perceived as missed opportunities, focus on what you did: You provided care, offered support, and loved your loved one unconditionally. These are acts worthy of acknowledgement and self-appreciation.

Another scenario: You might be plagued by regret for a disagreement or conflict with your loved one shortly before their death. The negative thought might be: **"If only I had handled that argument differently, our last interaction would have been more peaceful."** Again, challenge this thought. Relationships are inherently complex; disagreements are inevitable. While you might wish for a different outcome, that doesn't invalidate the totality of your relationship. Focus on the positive aspects of your connection, the memories of love and understanding. Remember that the desire for reconciliation is itself a testament to your love and remorse. Consider writing a letter to your loved one, expressing your feelings, seeking forgiveness, and acknowledging the impact of your actions. This can be a powerful act of self-healing.

Self-compassion practices, such as **mindfulness meditation**, can be invaluable in coping with guilt and regret. Mindfulness encourages you to observe your thoughts and emotions without judgment. When feelings of guilt arise, acknowledge their presence without getting swept away by them. Notice the physical sensations in your body – the tightness in your chest, the clenching of your jaw. Simply observe these sensations without trying to change them. This non-judgmental awareness allows you to create space between yourself and your emotions, reducing their intensity.

Guided meditations that focus on self-compassion can be particularly helpful. These meditations often involve repeating phrases of self-acceptance and encouragement, reminding yourself of your inherent worth and value. They may also include visualization exercises that involve imagining yourself enveloped in warmth, comfort, and support. These techniques help to cultivate a sense of self-acceptance and reduce self-criticism, which is essential for managing feelings of guilt and regret.

Furthermore, integrating self-compassion into your daily life can be beneficial. Practice acts of self-kindness, such as taking time for activities you enjoy, prioritizing your physical and mental well-being, and engaging in activities that bring you joy. **These acts of self-care are not selfish; they are crucial for maintaining your emotional resilience and fostering a sense of self-worth.**

Your worth and value are not diminished by your feeling of guilt or regret.

Remember that healing from grief is a journey, not a destination. There will be ups and downs, moments of clarity and moments of intense emotional pain. Be patient with yourself, acknowledging that the process takes time and that setbacks are normal.

Seek support from friends, family, support groups, or a therapist. These resources can provide invaluable guidance and support as you navigate this challenging period of your life. The path to healing from guilt and regret lies in self-compassion, acceptance, and the courage to challenge negative thought patterns.

Embrace the process and allow yourself the time and space to heal. Your worth and value are not diminished by your feelings of guilt or regret; they are inherent qualities that remain even in the midst of intense emotional pain you may be experiencing. **Through self-compassion and the application of CBT techniques, you can gradually lessen the burden of these emotions and begin to find peace.**

CHAPTER 13

Managing Sadness and Despair

S adness and despair are often the most prominent emotions experienced during grief. They can feel all-consuming, a heavy blanket smothering joy and hope. Unlike guilt and regret, which often involve self-blame, sadness and despair are more direct responses to the loss itself. They are the raw, visceral pain of absence, the aching void left behind by the death of a loved one. While these feelings are completely normal and understandable, their intensity can be overwhelming, leaving individuals feeling helpless and hopeless. The key to navigating this turbulent emotional landscape lies in a multifaceted approach that combines acceptance, healthy emotional expression, and the cultivation of supportive relationships.

Acceptance, in this context, does not mean resignation or giving up. It doesn't imply that you are happy about the pain; rather, it means acknowledging the reality of your emotions without judgment. It's about recognizing that sadness and despair are natural responses to loss, and that it's okay to feel them fully. Fighting these feelings only prolongs their grip, creating a sense of inner conflict that further exacerbates suffering. Instead, strive to observe your emotions as they arise without attempting to control or suppress them. Think of your emotions like waves in the ocean; they rise and fall, ebb and flow. Allow them to crest and crash, acknowledging their power without being swept away by them.

Mindfulness practices are instrumental in cultivating acceptance. Mindful breathing exercises, for instance, can help to anchor you in the present moment, reducing the intensity of overwhelming emotions. Focus on the sensation of your breath entering and leaving your body. Notice the rise and fall of your chest or abdomen. If your mind wanders, gently guide your attention back to your breath. This simple yet powerful technique can provide a sense of calm amidst emotional turmoil. Body scans, another mindfulness technique, involve systematically focusing on different parts of your body, noticing any sensations without judgment. This can help to ground you in the present and release physical tension associated with emotional distress.

Journaling can also be a valuable tool for cultivating acceptance. Writing down your thoughts and feelings can help to externalize them, providing a sense of distance and perspective. Don't worry about grammar or style; simply allow yourself to express whatever comes to mind. You might write about specific memories of your loved one, the emotions you are experiencing, or simply the thoughts that keep running through your head. This process can facilitate emotional processing and promote a sense of self-understanding. The act of writing itself can be therapeutic, providing a release valve for pent-up emotions.

Emotional expression, though often difficult, is crucial for healing. Suppressing your sadness and despair will only intensify their hold on you. Finding healthy and constructive ways to express your emotions can help to alleviate their intensity and promote emotional processing. Consider engaging in creative expression, such as painting, drawing, music, or writing poetry. These activities allow you to translate your emotions into a tangible form, providing a sense of control and accomplishment.

Talking about your feelings with a trusted friend, family member, or therapist can also be immensely helpful. Sharing your grief with others can reduce feelings of isolation and provide a sense of validation and support. Don't underestimate the power of simply expressing your emotions aloud; the act of voicing your pain can be incredibly cathartic. If you find it challenging to articulate your feelings, consider starting with simple statements like, "I'm feeling really sad today," or "I'm struggling with the loss of my loved one." Even these seemingly small steps can make a significant difference in easing emotional burden.

Seeking professional support from a therapist specializing in grief and loss is an important step to healing. A therapist can provide a safe and non-judgmental space for you to explore your feelings, develop coping mechanisms, and process your grief in a healthy way. They can also offer guidance on how to navigate specific challenges, such as dealing with difficult family dynamics or managing practical matters related to the loss. Remember that seeking professional help is a sign of strength, not weakness. It demonstrates your commitment to your own well-being and your willingness to seek support during a difficult time.

Social support is essential in navigating the depths of sadness and despair. Connection with others, even in the midst of overwhelming grief, can offer solace and a sense of belonging. This doesn't necessarily mean attending large social gatherings if you are not up for it; it can involve connecting with a close friend or family member for a quiet conversation or joining a grief support group where you can share your experiences with others who understand.

The shared experience of grief can be profoundly validating, reducing feelings of isolation and providing a sense of hope.

Support groups offer a safe space to express emotions without judgement and learn coping strategies from others. These groups provide a sense of community that can be invaluable during the grieving process.

Alongside **professional support and social connections, self-care practices are crucial for managing sadness and despair.** These practices are not about escaping from your emotions; they are about nurturing yourself during a difficult time. Prioritize activities that promote physical and mental well-being, such as regular exercise, healthy eating, sufficient sleep, and engaging in activities you enjoy. Even small acts of self-care, such as taking a warm bath, listening to calming music, or spending time in nature, can have a significant positive impact on your emotional state. Remember, nurturing your physical health helps improve your mental and emotional resilience. When overwhelmed with sadness, stepping away to engage in self-care, even for a brief period, can be a way to pause, reconnect with yourself, and return to navigate the emotions with more composure.

It's important to recognize that sadness and despair may fluctuate in intensity throughout the grieving process. There will be days when the pain feels unbearable, and other days when you feel a glimmer of hope or moments of relative peace. This fluctuation is a normal part of the grieving journey; it's not a sign that you are doing something wrong. Be patient with yourself and allow yourself time to heal. Remember, healing from grief is not a linear process; it is a journey with ups and downs.

The journey may be long and arduous, but with the right tools and support, you can find a way to live with your grief and honor the memory of your loved one in a healthy and meaningful way.

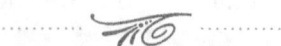

There will be days when the waves of grief crash over you, and there will be days when the waters are calmer. Learning to navigate these ebbs and flows is a testament to your strength and resilience. Self-compassion plays a critical role during this period. Treat yourself with the same kindness and understanding you would offer a friend going through a similar experience.

Managing sadness and despair during grief requires a multifaceted approach. **Acceptance, healthy emotional expression, strong social support, and self-care practices are all essential elements in the healing process. Remember that seeking professional support is a sign of strength, not weakness. With time, patience, and self-compassion, you can**

gradually navigate these challenging emotions and begin to find a path towards healing and peace.

The journey may be long and arduous, but with the right tools and support, you can find a way to live with your grief and honor the memory of your loved one in a healthy and meaningful way. The absence of your loved one leaves a void, but your life is not defined solely by this loss. You will find ways to cope, to live, and to honor their memory in a way that feels authentic and true to your own healing journey.

CHAPTER 14

Dealing With Anxiety and Fear

L osing my mother, father, and oldest son left me engulfed in a sorrow that words can barely capture. It wasn't just grief, it was a deep, lingering fear of the unknown. Their absence created a void that felt endless, and I often found myself gripped by anxiety so intense, it colored every part of my daily life. The future felt uncertain and overwhelming. I was afraid of moving forward without the pillars of love and familiarity that had shaped my world.

My father wasn't just a parent he was my best friend. We shared spontaneous road trips, private jokes during noisy family gatherings, and a mutual love for discovering new music. His presence grounded me. The thought of facing life's milestones without him graduations, weddings, even quiet weekends felt unbearable.

This fear was paralyzing. It wasn't just sadness; it was a constant ache, a sense of unease that settled deep in my soul. But with time, I realized that these intense emotions were a normal response to extraordinary loss. I also began to understand that while their physical presence was gone, their love had never left me.

I started to reframe my pain. I allowed myself to feel it, to sit with it, and slowly, I began to honor my loved ones by living not just existing. I found joy in remembering them: laughing at memories, keeping our traditions alive, and sharing their stories with others. I embraced healing through prayer, journaling, community, and acts of kindness.

Grief and joy began to co-exist. The ache remained, but so did a growing sense of peace. I now carry their love with me like a compass, guiding me through each step of life. And while I still miss them deeply, I've learned that even in the darkest moments, joy can be found not by forgetting, but by loving them forward into the life I continue to build.

Consider the technique **of mindful breathing,** but this time, not just focusing on the breath itself, but on its effect on your body. Notice how your chest rises and falls, how your abdomen expands and contracts. Pay attention to the subtle sensations – the coolness of the air entering your nostrils, the warmth of the air leaving your lungs. This heightened awareness of physical sensations grounds you, pulling your attention away from the swirling anxieties about the future. If your mind wanders, as it inevitably will, gently guide your attention back to your breath, acknowledging the thought without judgment, and returning your focus to the physical sensations of breathing.

Alongside mindful breathing, **body scans** can be extremely helpful. This technique systematically guides your attention through different parts of your body, noticing any physical sensations without judgment. Start with your toes, focusing on any tingling, warmth, or tension. Slowly move your attention upwards, through your feet, ankles, calves, and so on, until you've scanned your entire body. The process of consciously noticing and acknowledging these physical sensations helps to ground you in the present and can alleviate the physical manifestations of anxiety, such as muscle tension or a racing heart.

Another powerful mindfulness technique for managing anxiety is **engaging all your senses**. When anxiety strikes, focus intently on what you can see, hear, smell, taste, and touch. Notice the details of your surroundings – the color of the walls, the texture of your clothes, the sounds around you, even the subtle smells in the air.

This sensory awareness anchors you in the present moment, providing a powerful counterpoint to the anxiety-fueled preoccupation with the future. It's a way to reconnect with reality and interrupt the cycle of fear-based thoughts. This process helps to gently pull your attention away from the abstract fear of the unknown and back into the tangible experience of the present moment.

Beyond mindfulness, relaxation techniques like progressive muscle relaxation can significantly reduce anxiety. This technique involves systematically tensing and releasing different muscle groups in your body. Start with your toes, tensing them as tightly as you can for a few seconds, then releasing the tension and noticing the feeling of relaxation. Continue this process, moving up your body, tensing and releasing each muscle group in turn. This physical release of tension often translates into a reduction in mental anxiety. The act of focusing on the physical sensations of tension and release allows for a detachment from anxieties related to the future. This physical act creates a mental break from the obsessive thought patterns associated with fear and uncertainty.

Cognitive Reframing:
A Key Strategy for Managing Anxiety After Loss

One of the most effective strategies for managing anxiety related to grief and loss is cognitive reframing. This psychological tool helps individuals gain control over their thought patterns by shifting the way they interpret distressing situations.

Anxiety, particularly after the death of a loved one, often arises from catastrophic thinking—a mental habit where the mind fixates on worst-case scenarios and assumes they are not only possible but inevitable. These distorted thoughts can intensify feelings of helplessness and despair, especially when facing an uncertain future.

Cognitive reframing involves deliberately identifying these negative thoughts, challenging their validity, and replacing them with more realistic, balanced perspectives. It requires an intentional awareness that thoughts are not facts, and that perception can be reshaped to reduce emotional distress.

For instance, a common anxiety following the loss of a loved one may be related to financial insecurity. A person might think, *"I'll never be able to make ends meet. I'm doomed."* This thought is emotionally charged and rooted in fear, but not necessarily grounded in objective reality.

Using cognitive reframing, this thought can be examined:

- *Is it truly accurate to assume complete financial collapse?*
- *Are there steps I can take or resources I can access—such as community support, survivor benefits, or guidance from a financial advisor?*

By asking these questions, the individual can begin to shift their mindset to something more constructive, such as:

> *"This is a challenging time, but I am not powerless. There are actions I can take, and support systems I can rely on. I can work through this one step at a time."*

Through consistent practice, cognitive reframing can empower individuals to break the cycle of negative thinking, reduce anxiety, and foster a greater sense of emotional resilience in the face of loss.

Grounding techniques are especially helpful when dealing with overwhelming anxiety. These techniques focus on bringing your attention back to the present moment by engaging your senses, similar to what was previously discussed regarding mindfulness, but with a greater emphasis on a rapid and immediate response to an anxiety attack. If you feel an anxiety attack coming on, try these techniques:

The 5-4-3-2-1 method: Name five things you can see, four things you can touch, three things you can hear, two things you can smell, and one thing you can taste. This method brings you firmly back to the present moment by engaging all five senses.

Focus on your breath: Pay close attention to the sensation of your breath entering and leaving your body. Feel the rise and fall of your chest or abdomen. This simple technique can help to calm your nervous system and reduce the intensity of anxiety.

Hold an ice cube: The cold sensation of the ice cube on your skin can be a powerful grounding technique. Focus on the physical sensation of the cold as it registers in your body. This can quickly help interrupt catastrophic thoughts.

Physical activity: Engage in light exercise, such as a short walk or some stretching exercises. Physical activity can help to release endorphins, which have mood-boosting effects. It can also help disrupt negative thought patterns.

Listen to calming music: Putting on soothing music can help distract from negative thoughts and calm anxiety. Music can also induce a sense of comfort.

Remember that managing anxiety is an ongoing process, not a one-time fix. It requires consistent practice and patience. There will be days when anxiety feels overwhelming, and that's okay.

Acknowledge the feeling, practice your coping mechanisms, and know that you are not alone in your experience. Be kind to yourself, celebrate small victories, and continue seeking support when needed.

The uncertainty of the future after a significant loss is challenging, but with the right tools and support, you can build resilience, navigate your grief, and create a life that honors the memory of your loved one while cherishing your own well-being.

This is not about forgetting, but about adapting, growing, and finding your way forward. The grief will always be a part of your story, but it doesn't have to define your future.

The path may be winding and unclear, but with every mindful step, every practice of self-compassion, and every act of self-care, you're moving to a brighter, more hopeful tomorrow.

> This is not about forgetting, but about adapting, growing, and finding your way forward. The grief will always be a part of your story, but it doesn't have to define your future.

CHAPTER 15

Overcoming Isolation and Loneliness

The death of a loved one often shatters our sense of normalcy, leaving a void that extends beyond the emotional pain. This void often manifests as a profound sense of isolation and loneliness, a feeling of being adrift in a sea of grief, disconnected from the world and from ourselves. While the emotional turmoil of grief is undeniably challenging, the accompanying loneliness can be equally, if not more, debilitating. It can amplify feelings of helplessness, hopelessness, and despair, making the healing process feel impossibly arduous. But this isolation is not insurmountable. It is crucial to understand that your feelings are valid, that you are not alone in experiencing this profound sense of disconnect, and that there are pathways to rebuilding connection and finding solace in the company of others.

The first step in overcoming isolation is acknowledging its presence. Don't minimize your feelings or tell yourself you should be "over it" by now. Grief is a deeply personal journey, and the intensity and duration of loneliness vary greatly from person to person. Allow yourself to feel the pain of loneliness without judgment. This self-acceptance is the cornerstone of healing. Journaling can be a powerful tool in this process. Write down your feelings, your thoughts, your experiences of loneliness. This act of articulation can help you process your emotions and gain a clearer understanding of their source. Simply acknowledging the presence of loneliness is a significant step into mitigating its power.

Next, consider your existing social network. Who are the people in your life who offer support and understanding? These could be family members, friends, colleagues, or even neighbors. Reaching out to these individuals might feel daunting initially, but it's a vital step combating isolation. Don't feel pressured to engage in lengthy conversations or detailed explanations of your grief. A simple phone call, a text message, or even a brief visit can make a significant difference. Sharing your feelings, even just a little, can help alleviate the burden of carrying your grief alone. It can be incredibly comforting to know that someone cares and is willing to listen.

However, reaching out may not always be easy. You might feel hesitant, fearing that you will burden others with your sorrow, or that they won't understand your experience. These are valid concerns, but it is important to remember that most people genuinely care and want to help. If you're struggling to reach out, consider writing a short email or letter explaining how you're feeling. This allows you time to articulate your feelings without the pressure of immediate interaction. Sometimes, a written message can be more easily received and understood than a spontaneous conversation.

In addition to reconnecting with existing support systems, actively seeking new connections can be incredibly beneficial. **Consider joining a support group specifically designed for people grieving the loss of a loved one.** These groups provide a safe and supportive environment where individuals can share their experiences, learn coping mechanisms, and discover they're not alone in their struggle. These groups offer a powerful sense of community, a shared understanding that transcends the ordinary.

The shared experience of grief creates a unique bond, a mutual empathy that fosters healing. The knowledge that others are navigating similar challenges can be incredibly validating and empowering.

Beyond formal support groups, explore other social activities that interest you. Consider volunteering, joining a book club, taking a class, or participating in a hobby group. These activities offer opportunities to connect with like-minded individuals, engage in meaningful activities, and build new relationships. The focus on shared interests shifts the emphasis away from your grief, allowing you to experience a sense of normalcy and belonging. These new connections offer a welcome distraction from the all-consuming nature of grief, helping to broaden your perspective and foster a sense of purpose.

Remember that rebuilding social connections is a gradual process. Don't push yourself too hard or expect immediate results. Small steps are sufficient. Start with short interactions, gradually increasing the time and intensity of your social engagements. Be patient with yourself and allow yourself time to heal. There will be days when you feel more isolated than others, days when the weight of grief seems insurmountable. These are normal parts of the healing journey. On these days, focus on self-compassion. Be kind to yourself, acknowledge your feelings, and allow yourself to rest and recuperate.

Mindfulness practices can play a significant role in combating loneliness. By focusing on the present moment, you can reduce the intensity of ruminative thoughts that often fuel feelings of isolation. Practice mindful breathing, paying attention to the sensation of the air entering and leaving your body. Engage your senses, noticing the details of your surroundings – the colors, sounds, textures, and smells. These techniques anchor you in the present, interrupting the cycle of negative thoughts and promoting a sense of calm.

In addition to mindfulness, **engaging in activities that promote self-care is crucial. This could include exercise, healthy eating, spending time in nature, or pursuing creative hobbies.** These activities nourish your mind, body, and spirit, fostering resilience and a sense of self-worth. Remember, you are worthy of love and connection, and you deserve to prioritize your well-being during this difficult time. Taking care of yourself is not selfish; it's essential for your healing and for your ability to build new connections.

It's also crucial to recognize the role of self-compassion in overcoming loneliness. Be kind to yourself during this challenging period. Don't judge yourself for feeling isolated or for the pace of your healing. Grief is a complex emotion, and there is no right or wrong way to experience it. Allow yourself to grieve in your own time and in your own way. Avoid comparing your grief to others' experiences. Remember that every journey is unique, and there's no universal timeline for healing.

Finally, remember that seeking professional help is a sign of strength, not weakness. A therapist can provide a safe space to explore your feelings of loneliness, develop coping mechanisms, and navigate the complexities of grief. They can offer guidance and support as you rebuild your life and forge new connections. Don't hesitate to reach out for professional help if you feel overwhelmed or unable to cope with your feelings of isolation.

The path to overcoming isolation and loneliness after loss is not always straightforward. There will be ups and downs, moments of profound connection and moments of overwhelming loneliness. But by actively engaging in the strategies discussed – reconnecting with existing support networks, building new connections, practicing self-care, and seeking professional help when needed – you can gradually rebuild your sense of belonging, find solace in the company of others, and discover a renewed sense of purpose and hope.

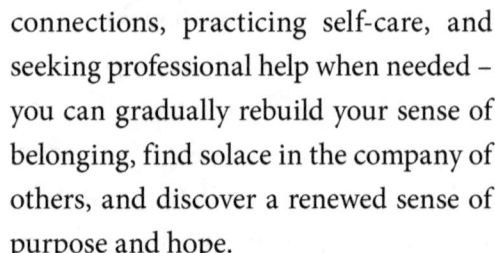

The healing process is about finding your own pace, acknowledging your feelings, and celebrating small victories along the way.

The journey may be challenging, but the destination – a life filled with connection and meaning – is worth pursuing. The healing process is about finding your own pace, acknowledging your feelings, and celebrating small victories along the way. It is a testament to your resilience, your strength, and your enduring capacity for connection.

Terrie on the left, with her daughter Jasmine, her
mom and dad, Larry and Sharon, her sons Antijuan
and Dominique, and her little brother, Quincy.

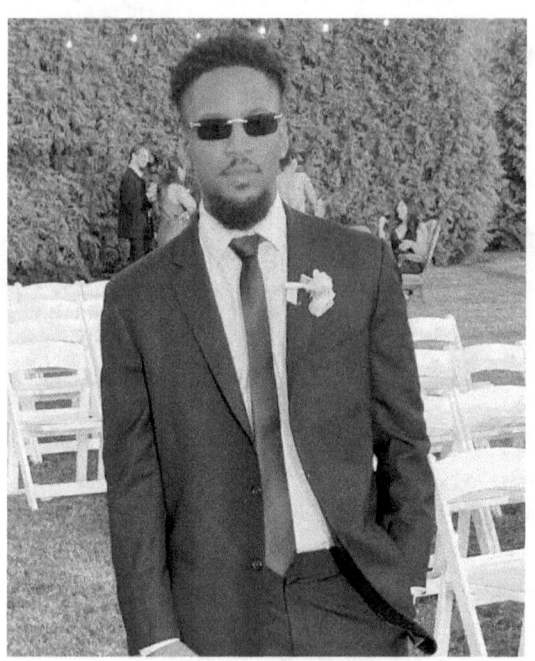

Terrie's son Justus

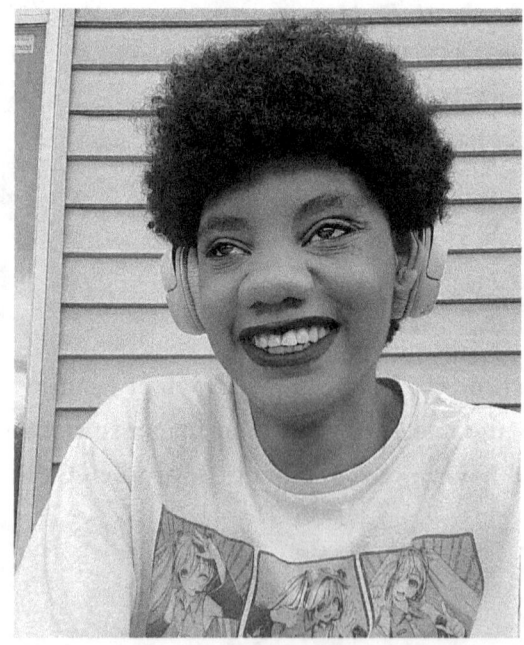

Terrie's daughter, Naomi

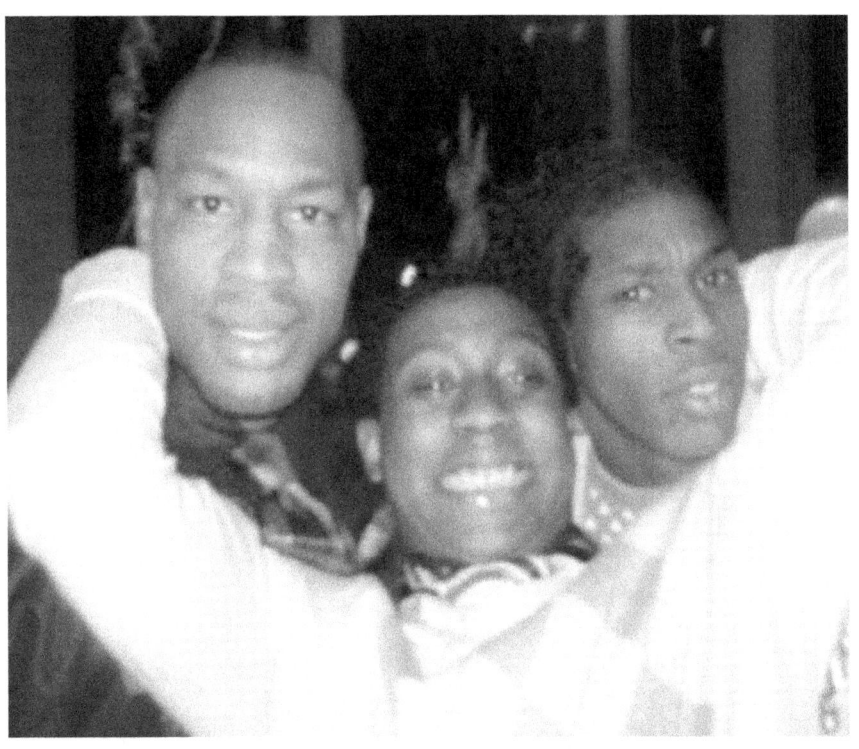

Terri's three sons: Ronte Eaton, Dominique Harris,
who passed away, and Antijuan Harris

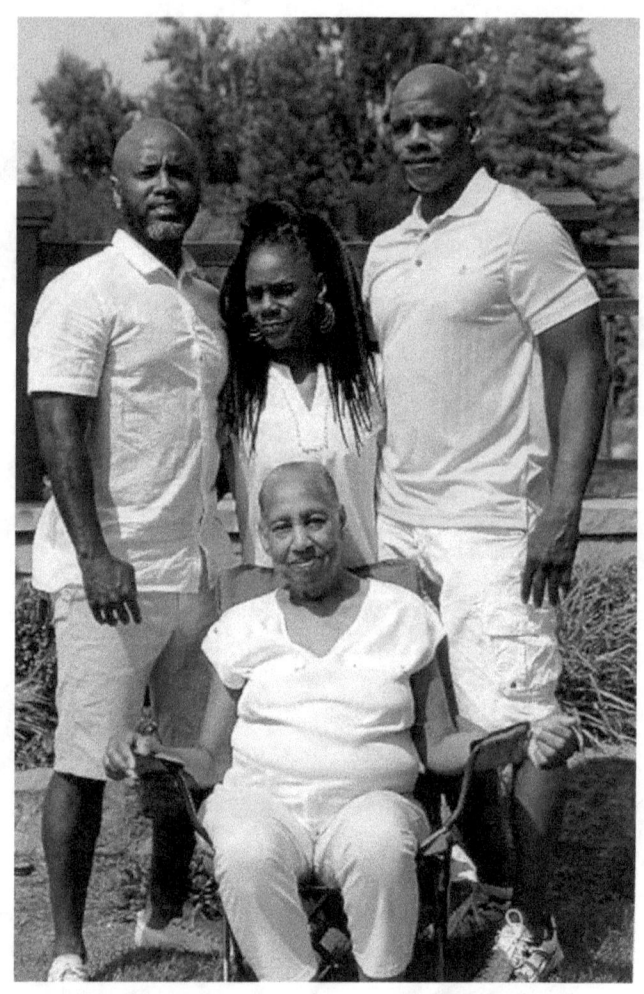

Terrie, Larry, Quincy, and Mother Sharon
who battled cancer for 30 years

CHAPTER 16

Finding Meaning in Loss

The profound sadness that follows loss often leaves a gaping hole, not just in our hearts but in the very fabric of our lives. The familiar rhythms and routines are disrupted, leaving us feeling adrift and uncertain. While the emotional pain of grief is undeniable, the subsequent search for meaning can be equally, if not more, challenging. This search is not a sign of weakness, but rather a testament to our inherent human need to find purpose and coherence in the face of adversity. It's a journey of rediscovery, a process of reconstructing our understanding of ourselves and the world around us in the absence of our loved one.

This quest for meaning often takes us on an unexpected path, one that may lead us to explore spiritual practices, revisit cherished memories, or redefine our values and priorities. It's a deeply personal journey, unique to each individual and shaped by their relationship with the deceased, their own spiritual beliefs, and their coping mechanisms. There's no single "right" way to find meaning after loss, and there's no predetermined timeline for this process. The path is winding, filled with moments of clarity and confusion, of hope and despair.

One powerful avenue for finding meaning lies in reflection on the life of the deceased. Taking the time to remember and honor their life is not simply an act of remembrance but a vital step in the healing process. It involves revisiting cherished memories, both the joyous and the challenging ones. Sharing stories with family and friends, looking through old photographs, rereading letters, or listening to favorite songs – these actions are not just nostalgic exercises; they are ways of keeping the memory of the deceased alive and weaving their essence into the tapestry of our own lives.

Consider creating a **memory book or scrapbook, filled with photos, mementos, and handwritten anecdotes.** This process itself can be incredibly therapeutic, allowing you to actively engage with your memories and process your emotions in a structured and meaningful way. You might find yourself reflecting on the lessons learned from your relationship with the deceased, appreciating the unique contributions they made to your life, and acknowledging the lasting impact they had on who you are today. This isn't simply about dwelling on the past; it's about integrating their legacy into your present and future.

One evening, I found myself clutching an old photo album, tears silently streaming down my face. I missed my mother, my father, and my son so deeply that it physically hurt. But as I turned the pages, I saw their lives not as lost but as *lived*. I began writing down memories, stories, lessons they taught me. I decided to create a memory book not just for myself, but for the next generation. In doing so, I realized that their legacy didn't end with their passing. It lived on through me. That gave me purpose to be the storyteller who keeps their light alive.

Spiritual practices, in their diverse forms, can offer solace and guidance in the search for meaning. For some, this might involve prayer, meditation, or attending religious services. These practices can provide a sense of connection to something larger than oneself, offering comfort, hope, and a framework for understanding loss within a broader spiritual context. The sense of community that often accompanies religious or spiritual gatherings can also be incredibly supportive, providing a space for shared grief and mutual support. It's important to note that spirituality doesn't necessarily require adherence to organized religion; it can encompass a wide range of beliefs and practices, from nature-based spirituality to mindfulness meditation to connecting with a higher power through personal reflection.

For those who find solace in nature, spending time outdoors can be a profoundly meaningful experience. The beauty and tranquility of the natural world can offer a sense of peace and perspective, reminding us of the cyclical nature of life and death. Walking in the woods, sitting by the ocean, or simply observing the changing seasons can provide a powerful connection to something beyond ourselves and can serve as a source of comfort and strength during this difficult time. Engaging your senses – the scent of pine needles, the sound of waves, the feel of the sun on your skin –anchors you in the present moment, offering a respite from the overwhelming emotions of grief.

There were mornings when getting out of bed felt impossible. The silence in the house, once filled with laughter and conversation, now echoed with absence. On one of those days, I decided to go outside—just for a moment. I stood in the sunlight, feeling it warm my skin. For the first time in weeks, I closed my eyes and breathed—not because I felt strong, but because something inside me whispered that I still had life left to live. That single step outside reminded me that healing doesn't begin with answers—it begins with *movement*, no matter how small.

Creative expression can also be a powerful tool for finding meaning. Through writing, painting, music, or any other creative pursuit, you can express your emotions, explore your thoughts, and process your grief in a constructive and cathartic manner. The act of creation itself can be deeply restorative, offering a sense of agency and control in a situation where much feels beyond your grasp. This creative output might take the form of a poem, a song, a painting, a sculpture, or even a journal entry that captures the essence of your experience, allowing you to externalize your internal world and find a new form of expression. This can be a way of honoring the memory of your loved one in a unique and personal way.

Volunteering or engaging in acts of service can also bring a renewed sense of purpose.

By directing your energy outward on others, you shift your focus from your own pain and find meaning in helping others. This can provide a sense of accomplishment and connection, countering the isolation that often accompanies grief. The act of giving back can create a powerful sense of purpose and instill a renewed sense of value and self-worth. It allows you to honor the memory of your loved one by embodying their values or by supporting a cause they were passionate about.

Give Yourself Permission to Feel Joy.

After months of barely leaving my home, I accepted an invitation to a family gathering. Guilt crept in when I laughed for the first time in a long time. I felt like I was betraying my grief. But someone pulled me aside and said, "They would *want* you to smile again." That moment helped me understand: joy and sorrow can coexist. Feeling joy didn't mean I had forgotten it meant I'm still capable of living. And in that realization, I found meaning in honoring their memory with *life,* not silence.

The search for meaning after loss is a journey characterized by ebbs and flows, moments of insight and periods of confusion.

The search for meaning after loss is always a progressive process; it's a journey characterized by ebbs and flows, moments of insight and periods of confusion. It's essential to allow yourself the time and space to explore these different avenues, to experiment with various approaches, and to find what resonates most deeply with you. There will be days when the pain feels overwhelming and the search for meaning seems insurmountable. On these days, practice self-compassion, acknowledge your feelings without judgment, and allow yourself the grace to grieve. Remember that the process of finding meaning is a deeply personal one, and there's no right or wrong way to navigate it. It's a testament to your strength, resilience, and enduring capacity to find purpose and hope amidst profound loss.

The path to finding meaning is often paved with unexpected discoveries. You may find yourself drawn to new interests, developing skills you never knew you possessed, or forging connections with people who support and understand your journey.

This evolution is a natural part of the healing process; it's a testament to your capacity for growth and adaptation. Embrace the changes, allow yourself to evolve, and trust that in time, you will find a new sense of purpose and direction in your life, one that honors the memory of your loved one while also celebrating your own continued journey.

This journey is not about replacing your loss but about integrating it into a richer, more meaningful life. The memories of your loved one will always be a part of you, but they will be woven into the vibrant tapestry of your life moving forward, adding depth, perspective, and a unique understanding of the preciousness of life itself. Finding meaning isn't about forgetting; it's about remembering, integrating, and creating a life that is both honoring and fulfilling. It is a testament to the enduring power of love, resilience, and the human spirit's innate capacity to find beauty even in the face of profound sorrow.

CHAPTER 17

Exploring Spirituality and Faith

For many, faith and spirituality provide a powerful framework for understanding and coping with grief. The inherent comfort found in religious or spiritual beliefs can offer solace during times of immense sorrow. This solace isn't solely about receiving answers to profound questions of existence and the afterlife; it's often about the sense of community, the rituals, and the established structures that provide a grounding force amidst the chaos of loss. The feeling of being part of something larger than oneself, connected to a divine being or a universal energy, can offer a profound sense of peace and acceptance.

The experience of grief varies widely depending on individual beliefs and the nature of one's faith. For some, religious rituals, such as funerals or memorial services, provide a structured path through the initial stages of mourning. These ceremonies offer a shared space for grief, allowing individuals to connect with their community and find comfort in shared experiences. The formal structure of prayer, hymns, and readings can provide a sense of order and stability in what might otherwise feel like a chaotic emotional landscape. These structured practices offer a tangible way to process emotions that might otherwise feel overwhelming and intangible.

For others, their faith offers a different kind of support. Daily prayer or meditation can provide a space for reflection and connection with a higher power. The act of prayer itself can be a source of comfort, offering a channel for expressing sorrow, seeking guidance, and finding peace. The belief in an afterlife or a divine plan can also provide a sense of hope and meaning, helping individuals to reconcile their loss within a larger spiritual context. This hope might stem from the belief in reunion with loved ones in the afterlife, or from a conviction that their loved one's spirit continues to live on in some form. This conviction can offer a sense of continuity and comfort, lessening the pain of finality.

It's essential to acknowledge that faith takes many forms. While some find solace in organized religion and its established practices, others find spiritual comfort in nature, mindfulness, or through personal reflection. For those who connect with nature, the natural world can provide a tangible link to the cyclical nature of life and death, offering a sense of continuity and peace. The quiet contemplation of the changing seasons, the vastness of the ocean, or the stillness of a forest can create a sense of awe and wonder, prompting reflection on the interconnectedness of all things and the ephemeral nature of life.

For those who find meaning through personal reflection, journaling can provide a valuable tool for processing emotions and gaining perspective. Writing about their experiences, feelings, and reflections can allow individuals to externalize their internal world, fostering self-awareness and deeper understanding. This self-reflection can lead to a greater understanding of their own spiritual beliefs and values, further enhancing their capacity for self-acceptance and resilience. Journaling is a profoundly personal act, offering a private space for exploring emotions and making sense of one's experience with loss.

It's also important to note that faith can be both a source of comfort and a source of struggle during grief. Some individuals may grapple with their faith, questioning their beliefs in the face of unimaginable loss. They might wrestle with feelings of anger, resentment, or abandonment toward a higher power. These are normal and valid responses to profound grief, and it's important to create space for these feelings without judgment. Seeking support from spiritual leaders, counselors, or supportive community members can be invaluable during these times of spiritual questioning.

These dialogues can lead to a deeper understanding of one's own faith, or they might prompt a re-evaluation of existing beliefs. The journey of faith is often a dynamic one, evolving and adapting in response to life's experiences, particularly those as profound as loss.

The process of questioning and redefining one's beliefs can be an integral part of healing and finding new meaning in life. It's not about abandoning faith but about allowing it to evolve and adapt in a way that resonates with one's current reality.

The role of spiritual leaders and community can also be critical during the grieving process. Clergy members, spiritual advisors, and faith-based support groups offer a structured and compassionate space for shared grief and mutual support. The shared experience of faith can create a powerful sense of community, providing individuals with a sense of belonging and understanding during a difficult time. These faith-based communities often offer rituals, ceremonies, and support networks designed to provide comfort, hope, and a sense of connection during bereavement. This sense of belonging can be especially important for individuals who are grappling with isolation or a lack of social support in their wider communities.

This journey of reconciliation, whether with one's faith, their inner self, or the world around them, is an essential part of the healing process.

In conclusion, the relationship between faith, spirituality, and grief is deeply personal and multifaceted. There is no one-size-fits-all approach, and it's essential to respect the diverse ways in which individuals find meaning and comfort during times of loss.

Whether through organized religion, personal reflection, mindfulness practices, or connection with nature, spirituality can offer a valuable source of support, guidance, and hope in navigating the complexities of grief. It's a pathway to finding resilience, acceptance, and a renewed sense of purpose in life, allowing the enduring legacy of love and faith to shine through even in the face of sorrow.

The search for meaning is often intertwined with the journey of faith, and respecting this intricate interplay is critical in providing holistic and compassionate support during the grieving process.

This journey of reconciliation, whether with one's faith, their inner self, or the world around them, is an essential part of the healing process. The path is unique to each individual and should be approached with empathy and understanding. It is in this exploration that true healing and renewed meaning can be discovered.

CHAPTER 18

Honoring Memories and Legacy

Honoring the memory of a loved one is a deeply personal and profoundly healing process. It's a way of acknowledging their life, celebrating their contributions, and keeping their spirit alive within our own hearts and the hearts of others. This isn't simply a matter of sentimentality; it's an active process of remembrance that can profoundly impact our own journey through grief. The ways we choose to honor the deceased often reflect their personality, our relationship with them, and our own evolving understanding of loss.

One powerful way to honor a departed loved one is through the creation of a lasting memorial. This doesn't necessarily mean an elaborate headstone or monument, although those certainly serve a purpose for many. A memorial can take many forms, reflecting the unique character of the individual and the memories you cherish.

For example, a family might choose to create a photo album, meticulously compiling images spanning their loved one's life, from childhood snapshots to recent family gatherings. Each photograph becomes a portal, transporting you back to specific moments, rekindling precious memories and strengthening the sense of connection. The process of curating the album itself can be a therapeutic act, allowing you to actively engage with your memories in a constructive way.

Including handwritten captions or anecdotes alongside the pictures adds a personal touch, making the album an even richer testament to their life.

Another deeply meaningful approach involves oral histories and storytelling. Gathering family members to share memories and anecdotes can create a powerful and lasting legacy. My family had the opportunity to have this as part of our Hospice plan, which involved interviewing family members about Mom and Dad's timeline. Family members told stories of them as individuals and stories of them as a married couple. This blessed our family, and we have a tangible legacy for future family members.

These shared narratives, perhaps transcribed and compiled into a book or even a digital archive, offer a vibrant and intimate portrait of the deceased, capturing their personality, relationships, and impact on others' lives. Such a collection becomes a treasured heirloom, passed down through generations, ensuring that their story and spirit live on. Other options might include planting a tree, establishing a scholarship in their name, or creating a dedicated space in the home filled with their belongings and mementos. The key is to choose a memorial that genuinely reflects the essence of the person you are remembering and provides comfort and solace to those left behind.

Alternatively, a memorial garden or the planting of a tree can be a beautiful and enduring tribute. The act of planting a sapling, nurturing its growth, and watching it flourish over time, can symbolize the enduring nature of love and memory, mirroring the cyclical nature of life and death. Choosing a tree that holds particular significance, perhaps one that resembled a beloved tree in their garden or a species they admired, adds a further layer of personal meaning. The garden or tree becomes a physical manifestation of their memory, a place of quiet reflection and remembrance, where you can connect with nature and find solace.

Another way to honor a memory is through the continuation of cherished traditions or activities. If your loved one enjoyed baking, perhaps you can continue that tradition, carrying on their recipes and sharing the joy of creating with others. This act not only honors their memory but also provides a tangible link to the past, grounding you in a sense of continuity. Similarly, if they were passionate about a particular hobby or activity, such as gardening, painting, or volunteering, continuing to engage in these activities can keep their spirit alive. This engagement doesn't just honor their passion; it also provides a creative outlet for your own grief, channeling your emotions into something positive and productive.

For those who were deeply involved in community life or philanthropic endeavors, continuing their work can serve as a powerful tribute. Volunteering for a cause that they championed, or making a donation in their name, is a meaningful way to extend their legacy and contribute to the world in a way that resonates with their values. This act of service allows you to connect with their spirit in a tangible way, carrying forward their commitment to making a positive impact. It also provides a sense of purpose and meaning in the midst of grief, directing your energies towards positive action.

In addition to these more substantial acts of remembrance, there are smaller, more intimate ways to honor a departed loved one.

Listening to their favorite music, watching their favorite movies, or rereading their favorite books can reconnect you with their personality and essence. These simple acts of engagement provide comfort and remind you of the joy and love they brought into your life. Preparing their favorite meal or visiting places that held significance for them can also be a profoundly personal way to maintain that connection. These smaller gestures, often performed in quiet moments of reflection, reinforce the feeling of their presence in your life, creating a sense of enduring connection.

Creating a dedicated space in your home to display photos, mementos, or treasured belongings can also serve as a powerful reminder of their life. This space doesn't have to be large or elaborate; a small shelf or corner, tastefully arranged, can create a comforting focal point. This designated area becomes a sanctuary, a place where you can go to quietly reflect, reminiscence, and feel connected to their memory. Adding personal touches, such as handwritten letters or small objects that evoke cherished memories, can imbue the space with a deeper sense of personal meaning.

The digital age also offers new ways to keep memories alive. Creating a digital memorial page or blog allows you to share memories, photos, and stories with others. This can foster a sense of community and shared remembrance, extending beyond immediate family and friends to reach a wider circle of people whose lives were touched by the deceased. These online tributes offer a platform for expressing grief and finding comfort in shared experiences.

Ultimately, honoring the memory of a loved one is a deeply personal journey. There's no right or wrong way to approach it. The key is to find what feels authentic and meaningful to you, allowing yourself to express your grief and celebrate their life in ways that resonate with your own heart. The process itself is a crucial part of the healing journey, providing opportunities for self-reflection, creative expression, and the strengthening of community bonds.

> Honoring the memory of a loved one is a deeply personal journey.

Through these acts of remembrance, we not only honor the deceased but also nurture our own emotional well-being, enriching our lives with the lasting legacy of love and shared memories. The process is fluid and ongoing; it's a testament to the enduring impact of the loved one on your life, a living tribute that grows and evolves over time. The key is to embrace the process, allowing it to guide you straight into a deeper understanding of both your loss and the enduring power of human connection.

This ongoing process of remembrance is not just about the past; it is about shaping the present and influencing the future, ensuring that their spirit continues to inspire and guide you on your life's journey. The legacy of love and kindness they left behind should continue to blossom in the lives of those they touched, a lasting tribute woven into the fabric of our lives. This is the essence of true and lasting remembrance – a celebration of life lived, a promise to cherish the memories, and a commitment to carrying forward their spirit in our own hearts and actions.

CHAPTER 19

Connecting With Nature for Healing

S pending time in nature can be a deeply restorative part of the healing journey after loss. Amid the chaos that grief can bring, the steady rhythms of the natural world—sunrises, changing seasons, the rustle of wind through trees offer a sense of grounding and gentle reassurance.

While grief often feels isolating and disorienting, nature provides a quiet refuge, a place where we can pause, breathe, and simply feel free. In that stillness, many find a renewed connection to themselves, a moment of peace, and the strength to begin putting the pieces of life back together.

Connecting with nature offers a profound pathway to healing after loss. The natural world, with its inherent rhythms and cycles, provides a powerful counterpoint to the often jarring disruptions grief inflicts upon our lives.

While grief often feels isolating and disorienting, nature provides a quiet refuge, a place where we can pause, breathe, and simply feel free.

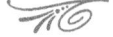

One of the most accessible ways to leverage nature's healing power is through **mindful engagement. This isn't about simply being *in***

nature; it's about being *present* in nature. It involves cultivating a deep awareness of your surroundings, tuning into the subtle details that often go unnoticed.

Start by choosing a location that feels peaceful and inviting. This could be a park, a forest, a beach, or even your own backyard. Find a comfortable spot where you can sit or lie down and simply allow yourself to be. Begin by focusing on your breath. Notice the gentle rise and fall of your chest or abdomen. As you breathe, become aware of the sensations in your body – the feeling of the ground beneath you, the temperature of the air on your skin, the weight of your body against the surface you're resting on. Slowly, begin to expand your awareness to encompass your surroundings. Listen to the sounds of nature – the rustling leaves, the chirping of birds, the gentle lapping of waves. Observe the colors, textures, and shapes of the natural world around you. Feel the sun's warmth on your skin, or the coolness of the shade.

As you engage your senses, allow yourself to simply be present without judgment. Don't try to analyze your feelings or force yourself to think about anything in particular. Simply observe the natural flow of your thoughts and emotions, allowing them to come and go without resistance. This mindful immersion in nature allows your mind to quiet, reducing the intensity of your grief and creating a space for inner peace. The rhythmic sounds of nature, the gentle breeze, and the expansive view can help soothe your nervous system, reducing stress hormones and promoting relaxation.

Beyond simple observation, you can incorporate active engagement with nature into your mindfulness practice. Gardening, for example, can be a deeply therapeutic activity. The act of nurturing plants, watching them grow and flourish, can symbolize the resilience of life and offer a sense of hope amidst grief. The physical act of tending to plants can be grounding, providing a tangible way to channel your emotions and redirect your energy to something positive. The repetitive motions of weeding, planting, and watering can be meditative, promoting a state of calm and focus. The vibrant colors and fragrances of flowers and herbs can uplift your spirits, offering a sensory experience that is both soothing and invigorating.

Similarly, walking in nature can be profoundly beneficial. Choose a path that suits your physical capabilities and allow yourself to move at your own pace. As you walk, pay attention to the sensations of your feet on the ground, the movement of your body, and the rhythm of your breath. Engage your senses – notice the sights, sounds, smells, and textures of your surroundings. Allow yourself to simply be in the moment without focusing on thoughts or worries. A leisurely walk in a natural setting can ease tension, reduce stress and anxiety, and promote a sense of calm.

Water offers a unique form of connection with nature. Whether it's the ocean, a lake, a river, or even a small stream, the movement of water is inherently calming and restorative. Sitting by a body of water, listening to the sound of the waves or the gentle flow of the current, can be deeply meditative. The rhythmic sounds of water have a natural tendency to slow down our heart rate and regulate our breathing. The vastness of the ocean, or the quiet tranquility of a small stream, can provide a sense of perspective, helping to put your grief in a larger context. The sight of water, whether calm or turbulent, can evoke feelings of both peace and strength.

Spending time in a forest offers a uniquely restorative experience. The scent of pine needles, the dappled sunlight filtering through the trees, the soft moss underfoot, all contribute to a sense of calm and well-being. The Japanese practice of *shinrin-yoku*, or forest bathing, emphasizes the therapeutic benefits of immersing oneself in the atmosphere of a forest. It involves slowly wandering through the woods, engaging all your senses, and allowing yourself to be completely present in the moment. Studies have shown that forest bathing can lower cortisol levels, reduce blood pressure, and boost the immune system.

Even if you have limited access to natural spaces, you can still incorporate nature into your daily routine. Keeping houseplants can bring the calming presence of nature into your home. The act of caring for plants can be therapeutic, providing a sense of purpose and accomplishment. The sight of greenery can be uplifting, and the fragrance of certain plants can be calming and restorative. Keeping a small garden, even a window box, can offer a similar therapeutic experience.

Creating a natural sanctuary in your home or garden can provide a dedicated space for reflection and relaxation. This could be as simple as a comfortable chair placed near a window with a view of nature or a small garden where you can tend to plants.

Incorporating natural elements, such as wood, stone, and plants, can create a calming atmosphere. The presence of nature in your immediate surroundings can promote a sense of peace and well-being, providing a respite from the stresses of daily life.

Nature's healing power is not limited to physical spaces; it can also be accessed through imagery and sounds. Listening to nature sounds, such as birdsong, flowing water, or rain, can be deeply relaxing and restorative. Using nature-themed artwork or photographs as visual aids during meditation can help to connect you to nature's calming energy, even when you are indoors.

Remember, the key to harnessing nature's healing potential is consistency. Make a conscious effort to incorporate nature into your daily routine, even if it's just for a few minutes each day. The cumulative effects of these small acts of connection can be significant, helping to restore your sense of peace, resilience, and well-being. The process is about fostering a deeper relationship with the natural world, allowing its rhythms and cycles to support your healing journey, transforming grief from a debilitating experience into a pathway of inner growth and a renewed appreciation for life's precious gifts.

The natural world is a constant source of renewal, offering solace, resilience, and perspective—essential ingredients for navigating the challenging terrain of loss and emerging stronger on the other side. The healing power of nature is not merely a suggestion but a powerful tool readily available to all who seek its restorative embrace. Engage it actively, patiently and consistently, and allow its inherent peace to permeate your being.

CHAPTER 20

Forgiveness and Letting Go

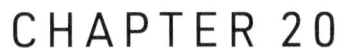

Forgiveness, in the context of grief, is not about condoning actions or erasing the pain of loss. Instead, it's about releasing the burden of resentment, anger, and guilt that can keep us tethered to the past, preventing us from moving forward. It's a process of internal liberation, freeing ourselves from the emotional chains that bind us to negativity and allowing space for healing and peace. This process, often challenging, is profoundly beneficial for our emotional and mental well-being. It's a gift we give ourselves, an act of self-compassion.

> Forgiveness, in the context of grief, is about releasing the burden of resentment, anger, and guilt that keep us tethered to the past.

The first step in this journey of forgiveness involves acknowledging the existence of these negative emotions. Suppressing or ignoring feelings of guilt, anger, or resentment only allows them to fester and grow stronger, casting a long shadow on our present and future. We must create a safe and accepting space within ourselves to examine these feelings without judgment.

Journaling can be an invaluable tool in this process. Writing down your thoughts and emotions, without censoring or editing, can help you identify the root causes of your pain and begin to understand their impact on your life. This process of self-reflection is crucial; it's the first step toward disentangling ourselves from the emotional knots that grief often creates.

Consider, for instance, **the common experience of survivors' guilt**. This intense feeling of guilt can surface after the loss of a loved one, particularly if we feel that we could have done something to prevent their passing. Perhaps we delayed seeking medical attention, missed an opportunity to express our love, or made a choice that, in hindsight, we deeply regret. This guilt can manifest as self-blame and self-recrimination, leading to overwhelming sadness and despair. Forgiveness in this context involves recognizing that, while we may carry regret, self-blame is counterproductive to healing. We cannot change the past, but we can choose to release the crippling burden of guilt by acknowledging our limitations and accepting that we did the best we could with the knowledge and resources we had at the time.

Forgiveness also extends to others.
Perhaps a loved one's actions, either before or after their death, contributed to the pain of the loss.

Maybe there were unresolved conflicts, hurtful words, or unmet expectations that still linger, fueling resentment and anger. Holding onto these negative feelings can only deepen our suffering.

Forgiving others doesn't mean forgetting or minimizing their actions. It means releasing the anger and resentment that these actions evoke and freeing yourself from the emotional prison of negativity. It is an act of self-preservation, recognizing that carrying the weight of another's actions only burdens ourselves further. This does not require reconciliation; it simply requires releasing your own emotional baggage.

One technique that can be helpful in this process is the practice of **compassionate understanding.** Try to see the situation from the other person's perspective. What might have been their motivations or intentions? Were they acting out of ignorance, fear, or pain?

Understanding, though not excusing, their behavior can help to lessen your resentment and foster empathy. It's crucial to remember that forgiveness is not a one-time event, but rather an ongoing process. It may involve multiple revisits to the emotions involved, and that's okay. The journey is what matters, not necessarily the immediate arrival at a state of complete forgiveness.

Letting go complements the process of forgiveness. It's about releasing the emotional attachments that prevent us from moving forward. It's not about forgetting the loved one or the circumstances of their passing but about freeing ourselves from the intense emotional grip of grief. This can involve various practices, such as mindfulness meditation, which can help us to become aware of our thoughts and emotions without judgment, thereby gradually loosening their hold on us. Spending time in nature, as discussed in the previous chapter, can also be immensely helpful, allowing us to connect with the natural rhythms of life and find solace in the world around us.

Therapeutic practices like Cognitive Behavioral Therapy (CBT) can be beneficial in addressing negative thought patterns and developing healthier coping mechanisms. CBT can help identify and challenge unhelpful thoughts that fuel grief and hinder healing. It provides structured techniques for managing these thoughts and replacing them with more balanced and realistic ones. This approach can significantly reduce the burden of self-blame and resentment, facilitating the process of letting go. Furthermore, through CBT, individuals learn to manage emotional responses more effectively, diminishing the impact of painful memories and paving the way for emotional recovery.

Art therapy can be another powerful tool. The process of creating art, whether painting, sculpting, or writing poetry, can offer a non-verbal way to express emotions that may be difficult to articulate verbally. It's a way to channel the intense feelings associated with grief into a creative outlet, providing a cathartic release and allowing for emotional processing. This can be particularly helpful for individuals who find it challenging to express themselves verbally.

Spiritual practices can offer a unique framework for forgiveness and letting go. For those with religious or spiritual beliefs, prayer, meditation, or participation in religious services can provide a sense of comfort, solace, and connection to something larger than themselves.

Writing this book felt intensely guilty. As I explored the stages of grief, I realized that if I'd understood and managed grief better while caring for my loved ones, I could have cherished our remaining time more fully instead of feeling numb and stuck.

Forgiveness and letting go, I now know, are deeply personal journeys requiring patience, self-compassion, and support. There's no timetable, and setbacks are inevitable. The crucial thing is to keep moving forward, gently, understandingly, one step at a time.

Professional help is always available – a therapist, counselor, or support group can offer invaluable guidance during this challenging process, "of which" I incorporate in my daily regime.

It's not about erasing the past, but about lessening its hold, moving forward with a lighter heart and renewed purpose. Allowing myself the time and space needed for healing will, I hope, lead to greater peace and acceptance. The harsh lessons of loss can become seeds of resilience and growth.

The path to healing is long and winding, but with patience, compassion, and persistent effort, inner peace and new meaning can emerge from profound loss. This journey of forgiveness and letting go is a testament to the human spirit's capacity for resilience, transformation, and finding profound inner peace, a peace I deeply need and strive for every day.

CHAPTER 21

Time Management for Caregivers

The emotional toll of caregiving is immense, often leaving little energy for self-care, let alone effective time management. Yet, structuring your time thoughtfully is crucial for maintaining your own well-being and effectively supporting your loved one.

The exhaustion that comes with constant caregiving can quickly lead to burnout, hindering both your ability to provide care and your capacity for emotional healing. Therefore, learning to prioritize tasks, delegate responsibilities, and utilize time-management techniques becomes not just a matter of efficiency but a necessity for your own survival and resilience.

One of the foundational principles of effective time management is prioritization. This involves identifying tasks that are essential versus those that are merely desirable. When dealing with the demands of caregiving, this can feel particularly challenging. Every task might seem urgent, every need pressing. However, a clear-headed assessment of priorities is vital.

Time Management for Caregivers:
A Guide to Balance and Well-Being

Caregiving can be one of the most meaningful roles a person fulfills—but it also comes with profound emotional, physical, and mental demands. The constant giving of time and energy often leaves little room for self-care. However, learning to manage your time effectively is not a luxury—it is essential for both your well-being and your ability to provide compassionate, sustainable care.

---

1. Understanding the Cost of Poor Time Management
Burnout is a real and serious risk for caregivers. Constant exhaustion without structured time can lead to:

- Reduced quality of care
- Emotional fatigue
- Increased health problems
- Loss of personal identity

Time management is not just about efficiency—
it's about survival, strength, and *resilience*.

---

2. Prioritization: What Matters Most Today?
When everything feels urgent, it's hard to know where to start. The key is to distinguish between **what must be done now** and **what can wait**.

The Eisenhower Matrix for Caregivers

Priority	Task Type	Examples	Action
1	Urgent & Important	Medication, medical appointments	Do immediately
2	Important, Not Urgent	Meal prep, scheduling respite care	Plan & prioritize
3	Urgent, Not Important	Non-essential calls, emails	Delegate/ postpone
4	Neither Urgent nor Important	Scrolling social media	Eliminate

💡 *Tip:* Skipping rest may feel productive, but over time, it drains your capacity to care.

---

3. Realistic Scheduling & Time Awareness

Avoid the trap of over-scheduling. Build in **buffer time** for delays and recovery. Remember:

- Be honest about how long tasks really take.
- Don't aim to "do it all"—aim to do what matters most.
- Use visual tools like planners, whiteboards, or digital calendars to map out your day.

🧠 *Mind shift:* Your schedule should reflect your energy, not just your responsibilities.

4. Delegation: You Don't Have to Do It Alone

Many caregivers carry everything on their own shoulders out of guilt or pride. But **delegation is a strength**.

- Ask family or friends to assist with grocery shopping, household chores, or errands.
- Hire professional support when possible (respite care, in-home aides, meal services).
- Communicate clearly—what the task is, what you need, and when.

💙 *Truth:* Accepting help protects your health and makes you a better caregiver.

---

5. Mindfulness: Reclaiming the Present Moment

Caregiving can make your mind race with worry and to-dos. Practicing **mindfulness** can help slow you down and calm anxiety.

- Start your day with 3–5 minutes of deep breathing.
- Take mindful walks or use guided meditation apps (like Calm or Headspace).
- Practice *compassionate self-talk* throughout your day.

🕊 *Reminder:* You deserve peace, even in the midst of responsibility.

---

6. Organization: Systems Save Time and Stress

Set up systems that simplify your daily routines:

- Use labeled folders or a binder for paperwork and medical information.
- Maintain a visible medication schedule or use a pill organizer.
- Try digital tools like **Google Calendar**, **Cozi Family Organizer**, or **Todoist**.

⚘ *Goal:* Reduce mental clutter to create more emotional space.

---

7. Make Self-Care Non-Negotiable

Self-care is not selfish—it's foundational. Just like a car needs fuel, *you* need physical, emotional, and spiritual replenishment.

Self-Care Essentials:

- **Rest:** Prioritize sleep and breaks.
- **Nutrition:** Plan balanced meals to support energy.
- **Movement:** Gentle stretching or walking boosts mood and health.
- **Joy:** Make time for what lights you up—music, art, nature, prayer, or connection.

🌿 *Mantra:* "Taking care of myself is part of taking care of you."

---

8. Be Kind to Yourself: It's a Process

There will be days when plans fall apart, when emotions overwhelm, and when exhaustion wins. That's okay.

- Celebrate small victories.
- Reassess and adapt without shame.
- Progress, not perfection, is the goal.

○ *Daily Reflection:* "What did I do well today? What can I let go of?"

In Summary: A Caregiver's Time Management Toolkit

- **Prioritize wisely.**
- **Schedule realistically.**
- **Delegate generously.**
- **Practice mindfulness.**
- **Stay organized.**
- **Honor your needs.**
- **Give yourself grace.**

Caregiving is not just a role—it's a journey of heart, endurance, and love. Time management allows you to walk that path with greater balance, clarity, and strength. You are not alone, and you deserve the same compassion you so freely give.

CHAPTER 22

Financial Planning and Resources

The emotional and physical demands of caregiving often overshadow the significant financial strain it places on individuals and families. The unexpected costs associated with medical care, medication, in-home assistance, and potential loss of income can quickly overwhelm even the most financially secure.

Before making these decisions during stages when loved ones are ill, make arrangements sooner. This is crucial for mitigating financial strain. Planning ahead allows for a more considered approach to budgeting and resource allocation. Before making these decisions during stages when loved ones are ill, make arrangements sooner. This section explores the financial realities of caregiving, offering practical strategies and pointing you to resources that can provide much-needed support during this challenging time.

One of the first steps is to honestly assess your current financial situation. This involves reviewing your income, expenses, savings, and any existing debt. Create a detailed budget, outlining all your income sources and meticulously tracking every expense related to caregiving. Many free budgeting apps and online tools can assist in this process, providing visual representations of your spending and offering insights into areas where you might be able to reduce costs.

Be honest with yourself about where your money is going; this detailed assessment is critical for developing a sustainable financial plan. Consider categorizing your expenses into essential needs (housing, food, utilities), caregiving-related expenses (medical bills, medication, home health aides), and discretionary spending. This will highlight areas where cost-cutting measures might be possible.

A significant portion of your expenses may be directly related to your loved one's care. This includes medical bills, prescription costs, therapy sessions, home health services, specialized equipment, and potential modifications to your home to accommodate their needs.

It's crucial to maintain detailed records of all these expenses, gathering receipts and statements for potential reimbursement or tax deductions. Many insurance policies cover portions of these expenses, but navigating the complexities of insurance claims can be a daunting task. Ensure you understand your coverage and proactively pursue all available reimbursements.

The unexpected loss of income is another significant financial challenge faced by many caregivers. If you have had to reduce your work hours or leave your job entirely to provide care, the resulting financial strain can be immense. Explore options for short-term disability benefits, unemployment insurance, or potential assistance from your employer. Many employers offer flexible work arrangements or leave policies to support employees in such situations; familiarize yourself with your company's policies and seek assistance from your human resources department. Do not hesitate to initiate these conversations; your employer may be more understanding and accommodating than you anticipate.

Beyond employment-based assistance, several government programs and non-profit organizations offer financial aid to caregivers. These programs often vary depending on location and eligibility criteria, so thorough research is essential.

Start by contacting your **local Area Agency on Aging (AAA).** AAAs serve as valuable resources, providing information about local programs, services, and financial assistance options available to caregivers. Their staff can guide you through the application process for relevant programs and assist in navigating the bureaucratic complexities.

Another crucial resource is the National Council on Aging (NCOA). The NCOA offers a wealth of information about financial assistance programs, including Medicare savings programs and other support initiatives for older adults and their caregivers. Their website contains detailed information, guides, and tools to help you find programs that fit your specific needs. Remember to utilize their online resources and contact their support lines; they are well-equipped to answer your questions and assist you in your search.

Navigating the profound emotional and physical demands of caregiving often obscures an equally significant, yet frequently overlooked, challenge: the substantial financial strain it places on individuals and families. The unexpected costs of medical care, medications, in-home support, and the potential reduction or loss of income can quickly become overwhelming, even for those with a strong financial foundation.

Proactive financial planning is crucial for mitigating this strain. Addressing these considerations early, ideally before a loved one's illness progresses significantly, allows for a more thoughtful and strategic approach to budgeting and resource allocation. This foresight can provide a much-needed sense of control and reduce future anxieties. This guide aims to illuminate the financial realities of caregiving, offering practical strategies and highlighting avenues for support to help you navigate this challenging journey with greater confidence.

One of the foundational steps is to compassionately and honestly assess your current financial situation. This involves a thorough review of your income, expenses, savings, and any existing debt. Creating a detailed budget, meticulously outlining all your income sources and tracking every expense related to caregiving, can be incredibly empowering. Many free budgeting apps and online tools are available to assist in this process, offering clear visual representations of your spending and insights into areas where you might be able to reduce costs. Being transparent with yourself about where your money is going is critical for developing a sustainable financial plan. Consider categorizing your expenses into essential needs (such as housing, food, and utilities), caregiving-related expenses (like medical bills, medication, and home health aides), and discretionary spending. This clear categorization will help highlight areas where thoughtful cost-cutting measures might be possible.

A significant portion of your expenses may be directly related to your loved one's care. This can encompass medical bills, prescription costs, therapy sessions, home health services, specialized equipment, and even necessary modifications to your home to accommodate their evolving needs. It is crucial to maintain detailed records of all these expenses, diligently gathering receipts and statements for potential reimbursement or tax deductions. While many insurance policies cover portions of these expenses, navigating the complexities of insurance claims can feel daunting. Ensure you thoroughly understand your coverage and proactively pursue all available reimbursements to alleviate your financial burden.

The unexpected loss of income represents another profound financial challenge faced by many caregivers. If you have had to reduce your work hours or leave your job entirely to provide care, the resulting financial strain can be immense. It is worth exploring options for short-term disability benefits, unemployment insurance, or potential assistance from your employer. Many employers offer flexible work arrangements or leave policies to support employees in such situations; familiarize yourself with your company's policies and do not hesitate to initiate these conversations with your human resources department. Your employer may be more understanding and accommodating than you anticipate.

Beyond employment-based assistance, a variety of government programs and non-profit organizations offer financial aid to caregivers. These programs often vary depending on your location and specific eligibility criteria, making thorough research essential. A valuable starting point is your local Area Agency on Aging (AAA). AAAs serve as vital community hubs, providing comprehensive information about local programs, services, and financial assistance options available to caregivers. Their knowledgeable staff can guide you through the application process for relevant programs and assist in navigating any bureaucratic complexities. Another crucial resource is the National Council on Aging (NCOA). The NCOA offers a wealth of information about financial assistance programs, including Medicare savings programs and other support initiatives for older adults and their caregivers. Their website provides detailed information, guides, and tools to help you find programs that fit your specific needs. Remember to utilize their online resources and contact their support lines; they are well-equipped to answer your questions and assist you in your search.

In addition to national organizations, consider exploring state and local government programs. Many states have programs specifically designed to provide financial assistance for long-term care, respite care, or other caregiving-related expenses. These programs may be need-based or targeted toward specific demographics; therefore, it is advisable to consult your state's social services department or health and human services agency. Their websites often provide comprehensive information on eligibility requirements and application procedures. Furthermore, numerous charitable organizations offer financial assistance and support to caregivers. These organizations frequently provide grants, scholarships, or other forms of financial aid to alleviate the burden of caregiving expenses. The Alzheimer's Association, for example, offers several financial assistance programs targeted at families affected by Alzheimer's disease. Similarly, organizations focusing on specific conditions or disabilities often provide resources for caregivers. Search for organizations dedicated to your loved one's condition to find potential financial aid programs tailored to your unique circumstances.

Beyond direct financial aid, exploring other avenues for reducing expenses is crucial. Consider negotiating medical bills, exploring cost-effective medication options through generic brands or discount programs, and seeking out less expensive alternatives to professional in-home care. This might involve leveraging support from family and friends, creating a structured caregiving schedule, or utilizing volunteer services. Even small reductions in expenses can collectively make a substantial difference in your financial well-being.

Managing your finances during a period of grief and caregiving can feel profoundly overwhelming. In such times, considering professional financial advice can be a wise step. A financial advisor can help you create a comprehensive financial plan, analyze your budget, explore potential tax deductions, and identify additional resources or support programs that align with your specific situation. They can offer objective guidance and help you navigate complex financial matters, thereby relieving some of the burden and empowering you to make informed decisions for your future.

**Remember, seeking help is a sign of strength, not weakness.
Caregiving is a demanding undertaking,
both emotionally and financially.**

The journey of caregiving is a marathon, not a sprint, and effective financial planning is an essential element for ensuring sustainable support for both you and your loved one throughout this journey. Utilize every available resource, advocate for your needs, and remember that you are not alone in this challenging experience.

Financial stability provides a crucial foundation for managing the other aspects of caregiving, allowing you to focus on providing emotional support and nurturing the relationship with your loved one while attending to your own well-being.

CHAPTER 23

Legal and Administrative Tasks

The emotional toll of grief is often compounded by the immediate and often overwhelming surge of legal and administrative tasks that follow the death of a loved one. Before making these decisions during stages when loved ones are ill, make arrangements sooner. This proactive approach can significantly ease the burden during an already difficult time.

This section aims to provide a clear, practical guide to navigating this complex landscape, offering support and direction during a time of profound loss. While the specifics will vary depending on individual circumstances and geographic location, the fundamental steps outlined below offer a framework for managing these essential matters.

One of the first priorities is locating and securing the deceased's will, if one exists. This document outlines the distribution of assets and designates an executor responsible for carrying out the instructions within the will. If no will is found, the process of estate administration falls under intestacy laws, which vary by jurisdiction.

Intestacy involves the court determining the distribution of assets according to pre-defined legal guidelines. In either case, it is crucial to immediately contact a solicitor or estate lawyer experienced in probate law. These legal professionals can guide you through the intricate legal processes, ensuring compliance with all relevant regulations and protecting your interests. They can help locate and interpret legal documents, and they'll act as your point of contact when dealing with official bodies.

The executor's responsibilities are multifaceted and demanding. They include gathering and inventorying all assets, paying outstanding debts and taxes, and finally distributing the remaining assets according to the will's provisions or intestacy laws. This process can be lengthy and involve numerous stakeholders.

Effective organization and meticulous record-keeping are paramount. Maintaining detailed logs of all transactions, communication, and expenses is critical, ensuring transparency and accountability throughout the estate administration. This detailed documentation will be invaluable when facing any potential challenges or inquiries. The executor is also responsible for notifying relevant parties, including banks, insurance companies, and government agencies, of the death. This notification triggers various processes, such as the closure of bank accounts and the initiation of insurance claims. A systematic approach, with a clear checklist and schedule, is highly recommended to manage these various tasks effectively.

Dealing with insurance policies is a crucial aspect of post-death administration. Life insurance policies, if held by the deceased, typically provide a death benefit payable to designated beneficiaries. It is important to locate all insurance policies, both life insurance and other policies like health, home, or auto insurance, and to immediately contact the respective insurance companies to report the death and initiate the claims process. This process usually involves submitting documentation, including a copy of the death certificate, the policy details, and potentially other relevant information as required by the insurance company. The claims process can vary significantly depending on the type of insurance and the specific policy details, and therefore, meticulous documentation is vital throughout this process. Be prepared to answer questions from the insurance company regarding the details of the death and related claims and keep records of all communication.

In addition to life insurance claims, the executor will also need to consider other insurance policies which may be relevant to the estate. This may include homeowner's insurance (to manage any claims related to the property after the death) or car insurance (which will need to be addressed immediately following the death).

It is essential that all policies are identified, and their coverage reviewed to determine potential benefits available for the beneficiaries. This thorough review will not only ensure you receive all the benefits to which you are entitled, it will also provide vital clarity around the estate's financial position following the death.

This understanding is vital for planning the management of the estate and will inform further decisions regarding asset management, debt repayment and final distribution of assets. Any ambiguity surrounding policy details should be resolved promptly through contact with the insurance provider and/or legal counsel.

Beyond insurance claims, the deceased's outstanding debts and taxes must be addressed. Debts may include mortgages, credit card balances, loans, and medical bills. The executor's responsibility is to identify and settle these debts using assets from the estate. If the assets are insufficient to cover all debts, the executor needs to be aware of the legal implications and seek expert legal guidance accordingly. Similarly, tax liabilities must be determined and settled. This often involves filing final income tax returns and dealing with inheritance taxes or estate taxes, depending on the size of the estate and applicable laws. The executor should engage a tax advisor or accountant specializing in estate taxes to ensure compliance with all tax regulations and to minimize the tax burden on the estate. Professional guidance is essential in navigating these complex legal and financial procedure and will assist with making sure everything is conducted efficiently and transparently.

The final stage involves the distribution of the remaining assets to the beneficiaries designated in the will, or according to the laws of intestacy if no will exists. This process demands meticulous record-keeping, ensuring that every transaction is transparent and documented. The executor should maintain detailed records of all distributions, including dates, amounts, and recipients. This meticulous record-keeping is crucial for accountability and will serve as evidence of the proper administration of the estate. It may also serve as a valuable record for reference for family members for years to come. Upon completing the distribution of the assets, the executor should file the necessary final paperwork with the court, concluding the estate administration process.

Navigating the legal and administrative tasks after a loss is undeniably challenging. The emotional weight of grief can make these practical matters even more daunting. However, a proactive and organized approach, coupled with the assistance of experienced legal and financial professionals, will ensure a smoother and more manageable process. Remember that seeking help is a sign of strength, not weakness. Utilize the resources available, whether they are legal professionals, financial advisors, or support groups, to guide you through this difficult period. The goal is not only to manage the practicalities but to do so in a way that respects your loved one's memory and allows you to begin the healing process.

Take each step systematically and allow yourself time to grieve while concurrently dealing with the essential administrative tasks that must be taken care of. The process may be lengthy and stressful but by following the advice in this section and seeking professional help when needed, you can navigate this complex period in a constructive way.

It is important to remember that you are not alone and many support networks are available to aid you through this process.

CHAPTER 24

Building a Self-Care Routine

T he emotional and logistical demands of navigating the aftermath of a loss can be profoundly draining. While the previous sections addressed the crucial legal and administrative tasks, this section emphasizes the equal, if not more important, necessity of prioritizing self-care. Grief is not a linear process, and the intensity of emotions can fluctuate significantly.

Building a robust self-care routine isn't about escaping grief; it's about equipping yourself with tools to navigate its complexities with greater resilience and self-compassion. A consistent self-care routine provides a foundation of stability amidst the chaos, enabling you to approach the challenges with a clearer mind and a gentler heart. Think of it as a lifeline, offering moments of respite and rejuvenation during a period of intense emotional upheaval.

Developing a self-care routine is a deeply personal journey. There's no one-size-fits-all approach; the ideal routine is one tailored to your individual needs, preferences, and circumstances. What works for one person may not work for another, and that is perfectly acceptable. The key is to experiment, discover what resonates with you, and adapt your routine as your needs change. This adaptability is crucial because the nature of grief shifts over time. What you find restorative today may not be as helpful tomorrow, and that is to be expected.

Consider what aspects of self-care resonate with you most. Some people find solace in physical activity, such as gentle walks in nature or yoga. Others find comfort in creative pursuits, like painting, writing, or playing music. Still, others find emotional nourishment in connecting with others, whether through support groups, conversations with friends and family, or engaging in community activities. The possibilities are vast and varied. Explore these different domains and select activities that nurture your physical, emotional, and spiritual well-being.

To build your personalized routine, start small, set realistic goals, and focus on incorporating one or two self-care practices into your daily life.

To begin building your personalized routine, start small. Set realistic goals, focusing on incorporating just one or two self-care practices into your daily life. For instance, you might commit to a 15-minute daily walk, practicing mindfulness for five minutes each morning, or listening to calming music for half an hour before bed. These seemingly small actions, when consistently practiced, can accumulate to significant positive effects on your overall well-being.

As you become more comfortable with these practices, gradually integrate additional activities into your routine. Remember, consistency is more important than intensity. It's better to engage in short, regular self-care practices than to attempt a sporadic, strenuous regimen that you're unlikely to sustain.

Consider scheduling your self-care activities into your calendar, treating them with the same importance as any other crucial appointment. This act of scheduling serves as a commitment, reinforcing your dedication to prioritizing your well-being. Even amidst the demands of managing estate affairs, make self-care appointments an unbreakable part of your schedule. Do not feel guilty for taking this time for yourself;

rather see it as an investment in your healing and ability to manage the other important aspects of the process.

Let's explore some examples of daily routines, keeping in mind that these are starting points and should be adapted to suit individual preferences.

Example Routine 1: The Mindful Morning

This routine focuses on starting the day with intention and calm.

7:00 AM: Wake up gently, without immediately checking your phone or emails. Take a few moments to simply breathe and appreciate the stillness of the morning.

7:15 AM: Engage in a gentle form of movement, such as stretching, yoga, or a short walk. Focus on the sensations in your body, paying attention to your breath.

7:45 AM: Practice mindfulness meditation, even for just five minutes. There are many guided meditations available online or through apps. Focus on your breath and let go of any judgment or expectations.

8:00 AM: Enjoy a healthy breakfast, savoring the flavors and textures of the food. Eat mindfully, without distractions.

8:30 AM: Journaling – reflect on your emotions, acknowledge your grief, and express your thoughts and feelings. This can be a powerful tool for processing emotions and promoting self-awareness.

Example Routine 2: The Creative Evening

This routine centers on unwinding and engaging in creative expression.

6:00 PM: Engage in a creative activity you enjoy, such as drawing, painting, writing, playing a musical instrument, or knitting. This can be a powerful way to express your emotions and find solace.

7:00 PM: Prepare a healthy and nourishing dinner. Pay attention to the process of cooking and enjoy the meal mindfully.

7:45 PM: Relax with a warm bath or shower, using aromatherapy oils or candles to create a calming atmosphere.

8:30 PM: Read a book or listen to calming music. Avoid screens for at least an hour before bedtime.

9:30 PM: Practice a relaxation technique such as progressive muscle relaxation or deep breathing exercises.

10:00 PM: Go to bed, aiming for seven to eight hours of sleep.

Example Routine 3: The Balanced Day

This routine incorporates a variety of self-care practices throughout the day.

7:00 AM: Start with a mindful 10-minute walk, appreciating the sights, sounds, and smells around you.

8:00 AM: Enjoy a healthy breakfast and listen to uplifting music.

12:00 PM: Take a break to practice a short, guided meditation (5-10 minutes). Use this as a moment to reconnect with yourself and refocus your energy.

5:00 PM: Engage in a physical activity, such as a yoga session or a brisk walk. Focus on the physical sensations and release tension.

7:00 PM: Spend quality time with loved ones or engage in a social activity. Connection with others can provide emotional support.

9:00 PM: Enjoy a warm herbal tea and read a book or listen to calming music.

10:00 PM: Practice a relaxation technique such as deep breathing before sleep.

These are just examples. The most effective self-care routine is one that's flexible, adaptable, and tailored to your unique needs and preferences. It is equally important to acknowledge that on some days, even sticking to a simplified version of your self-care routine may feel challenging. That is acceptable. On those days, focus on just one single act of self-compassion, even if it's just taking a few deep breaths or enjoying a warm cup of tea. The key is to be kind to yourself and to recognize that self-care is a journey, not a destination. Remember that progress, not perfection, is the goal.

Integrating mindfulness into your self-care routine can enhance its effectiveness. Mindfulness involves paying attention to the present moment without judgment. It's about observing your thoughts, feelings, and sensations without getting carried away by them. Mindful activities, such as meditation, yoga, or mindful walking, can help you connect with yourself, reduce stress, and improve emotional regulation. Even simple activities, such as eating or drinking, can be approached mindfully, enhancing your experience and fostering a deeper appreciation for the moment.

Remember, self-care is not selfish; it's essential. It's a necessary act of self-preservation, providing the strength and resilience you need to navigate the challenges of grief and loss. By consistently engaging in self-care activities, you're not only nurturing your own well-being, but you are also embracing the memory of your loved one by caring for yourself.

> Mindfulness involves paying attention to the present moment without judgement.

Prioritizing self-care allows you to grieve effectively, eventually allowing you to move forward and create a life that honors their memory while also allowing you to rebuild your own life. The journey of grief is unique to each individual, and building a solid self-care routine is a pivotal step in navigating this challenging and profound experience. It's an investment in your well-being, your healing, and your future.

CHAPTER 25

Maintaining Healthy Relationships

M aintaining healthy relationships during bereavement is often overlooked, yet it's a crucial aspect of navigating grief. The emotional toll of loss can strain even the strongest bonds, leading to misunderstandings and strained connections. However, nurturing existing relationships and cultivating new ones can significantly enhance your healing journey.

Open and honest communication is paramount. This doesn't mean you need to constantly talk about your grief, but rather, be upfront about your needs and limitations.

For instance, let your close friends and family know that you might need more time to respond to messages or that you may need to cancel social plans at short notice. Don't feel pressured to attend events or engage in activities that drain your energy. It's perfectly acceptable to say, "I love you, and I appreciate the invitation, but I don't think I'll be able to make it today. I'm still feeling quite fragile." Practice assertive communication; politely but firmly express your boundaries. This is not about pushing people away; rather, it is about protecting your emotional space so that you can manage your grief effectively.

Learning to say "no" is a powerful tool. It's okay to decline invitations or requests that feel overwhelming. A simple, "Thank you for thinking of me, but I need some time alone right now," is sufficient. Your loved ones who genuinely care will understand and respect your needs. Remember, it is not a reflection of your love for them, but rather a crucial step in your own self-preservation.

Some people might unintentionally offer unhelpful advice or make insensitive remarks. While their intentions may be good, these comments can be hurtful or invalidating. Learn to respond gently but firmly. For example, if someone says, "Just get over it," you could respond with, "I appreciate your concern, but grief is a complex process, and I'm working through it at my own pace." Remember, you are not obligated to justify your grief to anyone.

Similarly, you might encounter those who avoid mentioning your loss. This avoidance stems from discomfort or a fear of saying the wrong thing. However, their silence can feel isolating. Don't be afraid to initiate conversation about your loved one. Share memories, photos, or stories. This allows you to honor their memory and also allows your friends to continue their support for you.

Conversely, some individuals might become overly involved, pushing you to move on or minimizing your grief. Establish healthy boundaries with those who overstep your comfort zones. This might involve limiting contact or setting clear expectations about the type of support you need. It's essential to remember that you're not obligated to accept every suggestion, piece of advice, or gesture of support offered to you.

It is also crucial to communicate your needs with your colleagues. Let your supervisor or human resource department know if you'll need time off, adjustments to your workload, or flexibility in your work schedule. Your employer, in many cases, has a duty of care to your well-being and may be able to offer you support in navigating this difficult time. If possible, communicate with your colleagues as well – let them know that you may be less available than usual and may need some extra time to respond to emails or requests.

Maintaining a balance between expressing your grief and preserving your relationships requires finesse. While it's essential to be honest about your emotions, also understand that others may have their own limitations in processing your grief. They may not always know the right thing to say, and their attempts at offering support may sometimes fall short of your expectations. Extend grace and compassion to those around you, remembering that they are also navigating this challenging time in their way.

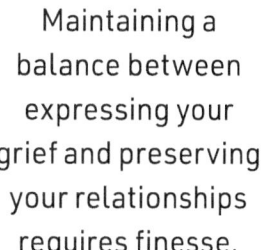

Maintaining a balance between expressing your grief and preserving your relationships requires finesse.

Building a support network is crucial. It's beneficial to lean on friends, family, and even professional support groups for guidance and emotional support. Connecting with others who understand what you're going through can provide a sense of validation and community, helping to alleviate feelings of isolation. Support groups provide a safe space to share your experience and learn coping mechanisms from others.

Moreover, engaging in activities that foster connection can prove incredibly beneficial. Consider volunteering your time to a cause that resonates with you. This offers an opportunity to give back to the community while also fostering a sense of purpose and connectedness. Alternatively, join a book club, take a class, or participate in hobbies that promote social interaction. This allows you to nurture new connections and expand your social circle beyond those immediately affected by your loss.

Remember that relationships evolve, and during times of grief, existing relationships may experience shifts. It's common to feel closer to some people while drifting away from others. This is part of the natural process of change and adaptation. Accept that your relationships might look different after the loss. Be open to letting go of relationships that are no longer serving you, creating space for new and more supportive connections to flourish.

Throughout this challenging period, prioritize self-compassion. Be patient with yourself and those around you. Acknowledge that communication will sometimes be imperfect. There will be misunderstandings, miscommunications, and moments of frustration. Yet, through empathy and a willingness to communicate openly and honestly, you can strengthen and maintain healthy relationships during your journey through grief.

Your relationships are a source of strength and healing, and it is important to actively cultivate them during this challenging time. It's a process, and even small acts of connection can make a significant difference in your overall well-being.

CHAPTER 26

Acceptance and Adaptation

Acceptance, a word often whispered with a sense of finality, is, in reality, a fluid process, a gradual unfolding rather than a single, definitive moment. It's not about erasing the pain of loss but about integrating it into the tapestry of your life. It's about acknowledging the irreversible nature of death while simultaneously finding a way to move forward. This involves recognizing the reality of your loss –not just intellectually, but viscerally, feeling the absence of your loved one in your daily life. It's acknowledging the void that remains, allowing yourself to experience the full spectrum of emotions that accompany it, without judgment. Resisting this process will only prolong the grieving period and hinder your capacity to heal.

This acceptance doesn't mean you suddenly feel okay about the loss. It means you've acknowledged its permanence and are beginning to find ways to navigate life in its presence. It's the difference between fighting against the current of grief and learning to swim with it. Imagine trying to swim upstream – exhausting, frustrating, and ultimately, unproductive. Instead, learn to adapt your strokes, your strategy, to work *with* the current. This is the essence of acceptance in grief.

Adaptation, the subsequent phase, involves restructuring your life to accommodate this new reality. This is not about replacing your loved one it is about adjusting to their absence. This could involve simple changes, such as rearranging furniture to eliminate the visual reminder of their presence, or far more significant adjustments, such as changing careers or moving to a new location. These adaptations may feel painful initially, but they are a crucial part of the healing process. They signal your capacity to rebuild your life, to create a new normal that incorporates both memory and hope.

For example, consider someone who lost their spouse. Adapting to life alone might involve learning to cook simple meals, manage finances independently, and tackle household repairs they previously relied on their partner for. This seemingly mundane adjustment is a powerful act of self-reliance and resilience. This isn't about forgetting the shared recipes or the collaborative approach to home maintenance; it's about learning to navigate these tasks alone, forging a new path forward while still carrying the memories of the past.

Another scenario might involve someone who lost a child. The sheer intensity of this grief necessitates a different kind of adaptation. It may involve seeking support groups, joining bereavement charities dedicated to supporting bereaved parents, engaging in memorial rituals, or even starting a foundation in their child's memory. These adaptations are deeply personal and serve as expressions of grief, love, and a way to give meaning to a life cut short. They aren't just ways to cope; they are creative acts of transformation, a testament to the enduring power of love even in the face of unimaginable loss.

The adaptation process extends to daily routines. Consider how you might adjust your morning coffee ritual. If your loved one used to make coffee, the silence of the morning may initially feel overwhelming. Instead of dwelling on the silence, make a conscious choice to adjust the ritual. Maybe you experiment with new types of coffee or create a new tradition, like listening to music while you prepare it. These small adaptations, almost imperceptible at first, signal a subtle shift – a movement away from what *was* to what *is*. They are the building blocks of a new life structure.

Adaptation isn't linear. There will be setbacks, moments of intense grief that bring you crashing back to the reality of your loss. This is perfectly normal. It's not a sign of failure, but rather an indicator of the depth of your feelings. These setbacks should not be viewed as obstacles, but as opportunities to reassess and readjust your coping mechanisms. It's like climbing a mountain; you might encounter storms and slips, but with perseverance and a renewed focus, you continue your ascent.

Mindfulness practices can be particularly helpful during this process. Paying attention to the present moment can help you ground yourself amidst the storm of grief. Simple mindfulness exercises, such as focusing on your breath or observing the sensations in your body, can help you regulate your emotions and manage overwhelming feelings. These techniques aren't about ignoring your grief; instead, they provide a space for processing your feelings without judgment. They offer a sense of stability and control in an inherently unstable situation.

Adaptation isn't linear. There will be setbacks, moments of intense grief that bring you crashing back to the reality of your loss.

One highly effective practice is mindful walking. Focus on the sensation of your feet on the ground, the rhythm of your breath, and the sights and sounds around you. This technique anchors you in the present moment, a counterpoint to the often overwhelming memories of the past and anxieties about the future.

Another valuable practice is mindful eating. Pay attention to the taste, texture, and smell of your food. Savor each bite slowly and deliberately, appreciating the nourishment it provides. This simple act helps you reconnect with your body and fosters a sense of self-care, which is vital for managing the emotional toll of grief.

Beyond mindfulness, engaging in activities that bring you joy, even if it feels forced initially, is crucial for adaptation. These activities might be ones you previously shared with your loved one, allowing you to honor their memory in a positive way. Or they could be entirely new pursuits, signifying your willingness to explore new aspects of yourself. The key is to discover activities that foster a sense of purpose and meaning, helping you redefine your sense of identity in the face of loss.

Perhaps you find solace in painting, gardening, or volunteering. These activities provide an outlet for your emotions, fostering a sense of connection and community, and reminding you of your own resilience. They are not simply distractions; they are investments in your future, affirmations of your capacity to find happiness and fulfillment even amidst grief.

Ultimately, acceptance and adaptation are intertwined processes. You gradually accept the reality of your loss as you adapt your life to the new circumstances. This is not a race; there's no timeline for grief. Be patient with yourself, honoring your own unique process.

**Embrace the imperfections, the setbacks,
and the moments of overwhelming sadness.**

These are all integral parts of healing.

Recognize that the path forward will be winding, filled with twists and turns. But with each step, however small, you are moving closer to a future where you can honor your loved one's memory while building a life filled with hope and resilience.

The journey is not about forgetting; it's about integrating, about weaving the threads of loss into the rich tapestry of your life, creating a new, meaningful narrative that incorporates both joy and sorrow, love and loss, past and present. This is the essence of moving forward with hope and resilience.

CHAPTER 27

Finding New Purpose and Meaning

The process of rebuilding your life after loss is not simply about coping; it's about actively creating a new narrative, a story that incorporates both the pain of the past and the promise of the future. Finding new purpose and meaning isn't about replacing what you've lost, but it's about enriching the tapestry of your life with new threads, vibrant colors that complement, rather than overshadow, the memories you hold dear. This involves a journey of self-discovery, a process of exploration and experimentation that can lead you to unexpected places and reveal hidden talents and passions.

One of the most powerful ways to find new meaning is through engaging in activities that bring you joy and a sense of accomplishment. This might involve rediscovering old hobbies that were put aside during the period of intense grief or exploring entirely new avenues of interest. Perhaps you always dreamt of learning to paint, play a musical instrument, or taking up pottery.

Now is the time to nurture those dormant passions, to allow yourself the space and freedom to explore them without judgment. The process itself, the act of learning and creating, can be incredibly therapeutic, providing a much-needed outlet for your emotions and a sense of purpose amidst the chaos.

Consider the therapeutic power of gardening. The act of nurturing plants, witnessing their growth and transformation, can be deeply symbolic of your own journey of healing and resilience. The connection to nature, the cycle of life and death mirrored in the garden, can provide a sense of grounding and peace. The quiet solitude of tending to your plants allows for introspection, for processing your grief without the pressure of external expectations. And the tangible results – the vibrant blooms, the bountiful harvest– offer a palpable sense of accomplishment, a testament to your capacity to create and nurture life amidst loss.

Similarly, volunteering can be a remarkably fulfilling way to discover new purpose. The act of giving back to your community, of helping others, shifts your focus outward, providing a much-needed counterpoint to the inward-focused nature of grief. It fosters a sense of connection and belonging, reminding you that you are not alone in your journey. Whether it's volunteering at a local animal shelter, working at a soup kitchen, or assisting with a community garden, the act of service can be incredibly empowering, renewing your sense of self-worth and providing a feeling of meaning and contribution.

One of the most powerful ways to find new meaning is through engaging in activities that bring you joy and a sense of accomplishment.

The act of giving back can also take more personal forms. Perhaps you can dedicate time to mentoring young people, sharing your skills and experiences to guide their paths. Or maybe you can use your talents to create something beautiful and meaningful – a quilt for a charity, a piece of artwork for a local exhibition, or a written piece reflecting on your experience of loss and healing. The possibilities are endless, limited only by your imagination and willingness to explore.

Remember that the pursuit of new meaning is not a race. There is no prescribed timeline or set of rules. Allow yourself the freedom to explore different activities, to experiment, and to discover what resonates with you on a deeply personal level. Some activities may initially feel forced or unconvincing but persevere. Give yourself time to settle into a new routine, to discover the joy and fulfillment that lie hidden within seemingly mundane tasks. The key is to approach the process with curiosity and openness, embracing the unexpected detours and unexpected discoveries along the way.

Beyond hobbies and volunteer work, consider the power of creative expression. Writing, painting, sculpting, music – all of these art forms offer an avenue for processing your grief, for giving voice to the emotions that may feel too overwhelming to articulate verbally. The creative process itself, the act of translating your emotions into a tangible form, can be deeply cathartic, allowing you to explore your feelings in a safe and constructive manner. The resulting artwork, whether it's a poem, a painting, or a song, can serve as a lasting testament to your journey of healing, a reminder of your resilience and capacity for growth.

Furthermore, consider revisiting old passions that may have fallen by the wayside before your loss. Perhaps you enjoyed hiking, photography, or cooking before grief consumed your time and energy. Reengaging in these activities, even in small doses, can provide a much-needed boost to your mood, helping you reconnect with a sense of self and joy. These familiar activities can feel comforting, offering a sense of continuity amidst the changes in your life. They remind you of your former self, of your strengths and passions, helping you to rebuild a sense of identity and purpose.

The process of finding new meaning is also deeply intertwined with the development of self-compassion. Be kind to yourself, particularly during the initial stages of this exploration. There will be days when you feel overwhelmed, when the grief feels too heavy to bear. On these days, allow yourself to rest, to give yourself permission to step back and avoid pushing yourself too hard. Self-compassion is not about ignoring your pain but about acknowledging your feelings with understanding and acceptance. It's about recognizing that you are doing the best you can in a challenging situation, and that your feelings are valid and deserving of compassion.

Engage in activities that nurture self-care. Prioritize your physical and emotional well-being through activities like exercise, meditation, healthy eating, and sufficient sleep. These seemingly simple acts of self-care are crucial for building resilience and coping with the emotional challenges of grief. They provide a foundation of strength from which you can launch into your exploration of new passions and purpose.

As you embark on this journey of self-discovery, remember that setbacks are inevitable. There will be days when you feel overwhelmed by grief, when the joy you find in your new activities feels fleeting and insignificant. These moments are a part of the process, reminders that the path to healing is not linear. Allow yourself to experience these feelings without judgment, recognizing them as temporary moments in a larger journey of growth and transformation.

Building resilience after loss requires consistent effort and self-compassion. It is a process of continuous learning, adapting, and evolving. Don't expect to find instant meaning and purpose; rather, embrace the gradual unfolding of your new narrative. Celebrate the small victories, acknowledge the challenges, and never stop believing in your capacity to create a fulfilling and meaningful life, even in the face of profound loss.

The journey toward finding new purpose is a testament to the strength of the human spirit, a demonstration of our inherent capacity for hope and resilience. It is a journey that, while undeniably challenging, ultimately leads to a richer, more meaningful life.

CHAPTER 28

Celebrating Life and Memories

C elebrating life and cherishing memories isn't about denying the pain of loss; it's about acknowledging its presence while simultaneously embracing the beauty and joy that still exists. It's a vital aspect of the healing process, a way of honoring the life that has ended while simultaneously affirming the life that continues. This involves actively creating spaces for remembering and celebrating, transforming grief into a catalyst for growth and appreciation.

One of the most effective ways to honor the memory of a loved one is by organizing a memorial celebration. This isn't merely a somber funeral; it's an opportunity to gather loved ones, share stories, laughter and tears, and collectively celebrate the unique life of the deceased. The structure of this celebration should reflect the personality and preferences of the individual being remembered. If they were vibrant and extroverted, the celebration might involve lively music, dancing, and shared meals. If they were quieter and introspective, a more intimate gathering with personal reflections and shared memories might be more fitting. The goal is to create a space where everyone feels comfortable expressing their feelings, sharing stories, and honoring the life lived.

Think beyond the traditional funeral service. Perhaps a picnic in their favorite park, a hike on a trail they loved, or a gathering at their beloved home. Consider incorporating elements that reflect their passions and hobbies. If they loved to garden, maybe the memorial could involve planting a tree or flowers in their memory. If they were an avid musician, live music or the playing of their favorite recordings could create a beautiful and fitting tribute. These personal touches elevate the memorial beyond a simple remembrance into a vibrant celebration of a unique life well lived.

The act of planning itself can be a deeply therapeutic process. It requires you to actively engage with memories, to sift through photos, letters, and mementos, prompting reflection and allowing for a deeper understanding of your relationship with the deceased.

The creation of a memory book or scrapbook is another powerful way to celebrate life and actively engage with the healing process. This isn't simply a chronological account of events; it's a curated collection of memories, emotions, and reflections. It's a chance to gather photos, letters, ticket stubs, and other memorabilia that represent shared moments and experiences. These tangible objects are more than just artifacts; they are touchstones, carrying the weight of emotions and memories that can be revisited and re-experienced. As you gather these items, you'll rediscover forgotten details, relive cherished moments, and unearth hidden gems of shared experiences.

Don't underestimate the power of writing. Compose letters to the deceased, expressing your feelings, sharing your memories, and asking unanswered questions. This can be an incredibly cathartic process, a way of processing your grief and maintaining a connection with your loved one even in their absence. Don't worry about creating perfect prose; just allow yourself to write freely and authentically, capturing the essence of your thoughts and emotions.

These letters will serve as powerful artifacts, bearing witness to your journey of grief and healing. They may become part of your memory book or scrapbook, or they may remain private treasures, to be revisited as needed.

Beyond tangible creations, consider the importance of storytelling.

Share your memories with others—family, friends, even strangers. These stories keep the memory of the deceased alive, ensuring that their impact on the world continues even after their passing. Sharing these stories allows you to connect with others who knew and loved them, creating a sense of shared community and mutual support. Each story shared becomes a piece of a collective mosaic, a beautiful and complex tribute to a life well-lived. The act of retelling stories provides opportunities for introspection, revisiting shared experiences, and solidifying the impact the person had on your life.

The power of expressing gratitude is intrinsically linked to celebrating life and memories. Take time to reflect on the positive aspects of your relationship with the deceased. Identify specific things you are grateful for – their support, their kindness, their sense of humor, their wisdom. Writing these things down, or sharing them with others, can transform the focus from loss to appreciation. Gratitude fosters a sense of positivity, softening the edges of grief and allowing you to see the beauty that remains.

> The power of expressing gratitude is intrinsically linked to celebrating life and memories.

Incorporating mindfulness practices into your celebration of life and memories can enhance the emotional impact and provide a sense of presence. Mindful moments of reflection, such as looking at photographs, reading letters, or listening to their favorite music, allows you to fully absorb the emotions and memories associated with those experiences. This isn't about passive observation; it's about actively engaging with the present moment, fully experiencing the sensations, emotions, and thoughts that arise.

Practicing mindfulness during the act of creating your memory book or writing letters allows you to focus on the process itself, rather than getting caught up in the broader context of grief. This heightened awareness strengthens the connection between you and the memories, fostering a deeper appreciation and a stronger sense of presence. The act of creating becomes a meditation of sorts, a focused journey of reflection and remembrance.

Furthermore, incorporating mindful movement, such as gentle yoga or a quiet walk in nature, can help to regulate emotions and promote a sense of calm. These practices allow you to ground yourself in the present moment, creating a space for processing emotions without getting overwhelmed by them. Mindful movement provides a physical outlet for emotional release, allowing you to experience the full spectrum of feelings associated with grief and loss without becoming lost in them. The physical act of moving your body serves as a counterpoint to the often immobile nature of grief.

Remember that the process of celebrating life and cherishing memories is ongoing. It's not a one-time event but a continuous practice. It's about weaving the life and legacy of the deceased into the fabric of your own ongoing life. It's about actively and lovingly remembering, finding beauty and strength in the shared experiences, and allowing those memories to shape your future.

The journey is not linear; there will be ups and downs, moments of intense emotion mixed with quiet reflection. Be patient with yourself, allow for the ebb and flow of emotions, and recognize that the process of celebrating life is an act of both remembrance and renewal. It's a journey of transformation, leading you to a place of acceptance, gratitude, and continued growth.

Embrace the richness of those memories, let them guide you, and allow the love you shared to continue to nurture and sustain you. The act of remembering becomes an act of living, a testament to the enduring power of love and connection. And through this process, you will not only honor their memory, but you will also find strength and resilience within yourself.

CHAPTER 29

Cultivating Self-Compassion and Forgiveness

T he journey through grief is rarely a straightforward path. It's a winding road, filled with unexpected turns and emotional detours. While celebrating life and cherishing memories is a crucial part of the healing process, it's equally important to acknowledge the internal landscape of your experience. This involves cultivating self-compassion and extending forgiveness—both to yourself and to others involved in the loss. These are not merely platitudes; they are active, vital components of emotional recovery and the development of resilience.

Self-compassion, often misunderstood as self-indulgence, is actually a powerful antidote to the harsh self-criticism that often accompanies grief. When loss strikes, it's common to engage in negative self-talk, to berate ourselves for past actions or inactions, for words left unsaid, or opportunities missed. We may replay moments, analyzing them with a critical eye, searching for flaws and failures. This self-flagellation only deepens the pain, hindering the healing process. Self-compassion, on the other hand, involves treating yourself with the same kindness, understanding, and patience you would offer a close friend facing a similar situation.

Imagine a friend sharing their grief with you. Would you berate them for their perceived shortcomings? Probably not. Instead, you would likely offer words of comfort, empathy, and reassurance. You would acknowledge their pain, validate their feelings, and remind them of their strengths and resilience. This is the essence of self-compassion—extending that same kindness and understanding to yourself.

Several practices can help cultivate self-compassion. Mindfulness meditation, for instance, is a powerful tool for observing your thoughts and feelings without judgment. When negative self-talk arises—the familiar chorus of "should haves" and "could haves"—simply acknowledge it without getting swept away by it. Notice the thoughts as they arise, like clouds passing in the sky, allowing them to drift by without clinging to them.

Another valuable practice is self-compassionate journaling. Write down your thoughts and feelings without censoring yourself. Allow yourself to express your anger, sadness, guilt, or regret without judgment. Once you have poured out your emotions onto the page, try reframing your negative self-talk with more compassionate and understanding language. Instead of saying, "I should have done this differently," try, "I did the best I could with the information and resources I had at the time." This simple shift in language can make a significant difference in your internal experience.

Beyond journaling and meditation, consider engaging in acts of self-care. These are not selfish indulgences; they are essential acts of self-compassion. Engage in activities that bring you joy and comfort—reading a book, listening to music, spending time in nature, or pursuing a hobby. These activities provide a much-needed respite from the intensity of grief, allowing you to replenish your emotional reserves and build resilience.

Forgiveness, another vital element of the healing journey, is often the most challenging. It may involve forgiving yourself for perceived failures or shortcomings, or it may involve forgiving others involved in the loss. This doesn't necessarily mean condoning harmful actions or minimizing the pain caused. Rather, it means releasing the resentment and anger that can consume you, preventing you from moving forward.

Forgiving yourself can be particularly difficult. You may carry a burden of guilt or regret, replaying past events and agonizing over what you could have done differently. Remember that self-blame is a common response to loss, but it is rarely productive. It's crucial to recognize that you are not responsible for everything that happens in life. Accepting that there are things beyond your control is a vital step towards self-forgiveness.

The process of forgiveness is not a single event but a continuous practice. It's a journey, not a destination. It may involve writing letters to yourself or to others, expressing your feelings and seeking understanding. It may involve engaging in compassionate dialogue with yourself, acknowledging your pain and validating your experience. It may involve seeking professional support from a therapist or counselor who can guide you through the process.

Forgiving others involved in the loss can be even more challenging. This might include family members, friends, or even medical professionals. Resentment, anger, and even blame may arise, clouding your judgment and hindering your healing. While it's important to acknowledge your feelings and validate your experience, holding onto these negative emotions will only prolong your suffering.

Forgiveness doesn't necessarily mean reconciling with those you hold responsible. It simply means releasing the emotional burden you are carrying. This can be achieved through various practices, such as writing letters expressing your feelings, engaging in mindful reflection, or seeking professional guidance. Consider the benefit of releasing the anger; the energy spent on resentment could be redirected towards healing and self-care.

Remember that forgiveness is a process, not a destination. It's a gradual letting go, a release of the burden you carry. It is not about minimizing the harm caused or condoning the actions of others. It is about freeing yourself from the chains of resentment and allowing yourself to move forward.

Integrating self-compassion and forgiveness into your healing journey requires patience and perseverance. It's not a quick fix but a gradual transformation. There will be setbacks and moments of relapse, times when the old patterns of self-criticism and resentment resurface.

This journey, though challenging, ultimately leads to a deeper understanding of yourself and a greater capacity for empathy and compassion.

Be kind to yourself during these moments; acknowledge your experience and gently redirect your focus back to self-compassion and forgiveness.

Recognize that the journey through grief is unique to each individual. There is no right or wrong way to feel or heal. Be patient with yourself and celebrate the small victories along the way. Cultivating self-compassion and extending forgiveness are powerful tools that can empower you to move forward with hope and resilience, transforming grief into a catalyst for growth and personal transformation.

This journey, though challenging, ultimately leads to a deeper understanding of yourself and a greater capacity for empathy and compassion. The resilience you cultivate during this process will serve you throughout your life, strengthening your ability to navigate future challenges with grace and fortitude. The pain of loss will always be a part of your story, but it will no longer define you.

CHAPTER 30

Hope for the Future

The journey through grief, as we've explored, is deeply personal and multifaceted. It's a process of navigating intense emotions, confronting difficult truths, and ultimately, finding a way to live with the loss. While the pain may linger, and the memories may remain vivid, it's crucial to remember that healing is possible. A fulfilling and meaningful life can be built even after experiencing profound loss. This isn't about forgetting or erasing the past; it's about integrating the experience into the tapestry of your life, allowing it to shape your future rather than define it.

Cultivating hope in the aftermath of grief isn't about denying the pain pretending it doesn't exist. It's about acknowledging the depth of your sorrow while simultaneously nurturing a belief in the possibility of future joy, meaning, and connection. It's about finding the courage to look to the horizon, even when the path ahead seems shrouded in uncertainty.

One of the most effective ways to cultivate hope is through mindfulness. By practicing mindfulness, we learn to focus on the present moment rather than dwelling on the past or anxiously anticipating the future. This doesn't mean ignoring difficult emotions; instead, it means observing them without judgment, acknowledging their presence without being overwhelmed by them.

Through mindfulness meditation, for instance, you can learn to gently guide your attention back to the breath, to the sensations in your body, to the sounds around you, whenever your thoughts wander to painful memories or anxieties about the future. This practice helps create space between you and your thoughts and emotions, allowing you to experience them with greater clarity and less intensity.

Incorporating self-care practices into your daily routine is another essential step in nurturing hope. Self-care, in this context, isn't about indulging in luxuries; it's about engaging in activities that nourish your physical, emotional, and spiritual well-being. This might involve regular exercise, healthy eating, getting sufficient sleep, spending time in nature, engaging in creative pursuits, or simply taking time each day to relax and rejuvenate. These seemingly small acts of self-compassion can have a profound impact on your overall mood and resilience.

Connecting with others is also crucial for fostering hope. Sharing your grief with trusted friends, family members, or support groups can provide a sense of connection and belonging, reminding you that you are not alone in your pain. These connections offer opportunities for mutual support, shared understanding, and the validation of your feelings. It's important to seek out individuals who offer genuine empathy and understanding, who can listen without judgment and offer a safe space for you to express your emotions. Avoid those who minimize your experience or offer unsolicited advice that feels invalidating.

Engaging in meaningful activities can also help rekindle hope. This might involve returning to hobbies you previously enjoyed, pursuing new interests, volunteering your time to a cause you care about, or connecting with your community. These activities not only offer a distraction from grief but also provide a sense of purpose and accomplishment, helping to restore a sense of meaning and direction in your life.

Consider setting realistic goals for the future. These goals don't have to be grand or ambitious; they can be small, achievable steps that move you in a more hopeful and fulfilling future. For example, you might set a goal to walk for 30 minutes each day, to read a book each week, or to connect with a friend once a week. Achieving these small victories can build momentum and reinforce your belief in your ability to move forward.

Remember that the path to healing is not linear. There will be days when you feel overwhelmed by grief, days when the pain feels unbearable. This is a normal part of the grieving process. Be patient with yourself, acknowledge your feelings, and allow yourself to grieve without judgment. Don't expect to "get over" your loss; instead, focus on learning to live with it, to integrate it into your life story, and to find meaning and purpose despite the pain.

> Hope is not a passive state; it is an active process.

It's also important to recognize that hope is not a passive state; it is an active process. It requires conscious effort, dedication, and self-compassion. It demands that you actively seek out opportunities for joy, connection, and meaning. It requires you to cultivate a belief in your own resilience and your capacity to overcome adversity.

Forgiveness, as discussed earlier, plays a vital role in fostering hope.

Forgiving yourself for perceived shortcomings or mistakes, and forgiving others involved in your loss, is not about condoning harmful actions but about releasing the burden of resentment and anger that can hinder your healing. This doesn't mean forgetting or minimizing the pain; it means freeing yourself from the emotional chains of the past so you can move forward with a lighter heart and a clearer mind.

Consider seeking professional support if you are struggling to cope with your grief. A therapist or counselor can provide guidance, support, and tools to help you navigate your emotions and develop healthy coping mechanisms. They can offer a safe and non-judgmental space for you to explore your feelings and develop strategies for moving forward. Don't hesitate to reach out for help if you need it; seeking professional support is a sign of strength, not weakness.

The future holds uncertainty, yes, but it also holds possibility. The capacity for joy, connection, and meaning remains, even after profound loss. By cultivating hope, practicing self-compassion, and fostering resilience, you can navigate the challenging terrain of grief and emerge stronger, wiser, and more compassionate. Your journey will be unique to you, but the destination – a life filled with purpose and meaning – is within reach.

Remember the importance of celebrating small victories. Acknowledge your progress, however small it may seem. Each step forward, each act of self-care, each moment of connection with others, is a testament to your resilience and your capacity for healing. These seemingly insignificant moments accumulate, creating a powerful current that carries you into a brighter future.

The path to hope isn't paved with easy answers or quick fixes. It's a winding road with its share of ups and downs, twists and turns.

There will be days when you feel discouraged, days when the weight of your grief feels overwhelming. But these moments are not indicators of failure; they are a normal part of the healing process. Recognize them, acknowledge them, and then gently redirect your attention back to self-compassion, connection, and the cultivation of hope.

Finally, remember that grief is a transformative experience. It changes you, shapes you, and deepens your understanding of life's fragility and beauty. While the pain of loss may never completely disappear, it can evolve over time, becoming a source of wisdom, empathy, and resilience.

The future may hold challenges, but it also holds opportunities for growth, connection, and a renewed sense of purpose. Embrace the journey, celebrate the small victories, and never lose sight of the hope that resides within you, waiting to be nurtured and allowed to flourish. The future, although uncertain, holds the potential for a life filled with meaning, joy, and lasting peace. Allow yourself the time and space to discover it.

ACKNOWLEDGEMENTS

Thank you to my Children: Ronte, Antjuan, Jasmine, Justus, Naomi, MyLisha, Mylissa, Sharnice, Namia, Tyra, and all my grandchildren. My Brothers: Larry Harris Jr, and Quincy Harris.

Thanks to Jennifer Harris.

Thanks to my Aunties, Uncles, and Cousins who all played a role in the development of this book.

To Dr. and Mrs. Montgomery who preciously cared for my parents and have always been a support. Thank you.

Thank you to every single Medical Doctor, Nurse, and First Responder, and to the Department Of Veterans Affairs and VA Hospitals

Writing this book has been a deeply rewarding experience, and I am immensely grateful to the many individuals who contributed to its creation.

I want to thank my editor, Mary Ethel Eckard, for her insightful guidance, unwavering support, and belief in this project. Her expertise and encouragement have been invaluable throughout the editing and publishing process.

I extend my sincere gratitude to the individuals who shared their personal stories of grief and resilience. Their vulnerability and willingness to share their experiences have profoundly enriched this book and given it a powerful, authentic voice. Their courage in facing their pain and their commitment to healing served as a constant source of inspiration.

I thank my friends for their patience, understanding, and support during this endeavor. Your love and encouragement provided the strength and motivation necessary to complete this work.

GLOSSARY

Bereavement: The state of having suffered a loss, typically through death.

Complicated Grief: A type of grief that is unusually prolonged or intense, interfering significantly with daily life.

Grief: The emotional response to loss, often characterized by sadness, anger, guilt, and acceptance.

Hope: A feeling of expectation and desire for a certain thing to happen.

Mindfulness: The practice of paying attention to the present moment without judgment.

Mourning: The process of adapting to loss, often involving rituals and practices.

Resilience: The ability to recover quickly from difficulties.

Self-compassion: Treating oneself with kindness, understanding, and acceptance.

Trauma: A deeply distressing or disturbing experience.

APPENDIX

https://www.mayoclinic.org/tests-procedures/cognitive-behavioral
-therapy/about/pac-20384610

https://www.apa.org/ptsd-guideline/patients-and-families/
cognitive-behavioral

https://mhanational.org/resources/maintaining-boundaries-as-
a-caregiver-go-from-guilt-to-glow/

https://athomeindependentliving.com/learning-to-say-no-as-a-
caregiver/

https://mhanational.org/resources/maintaining-boundaries-as-
a-caregiver-go-from-guilt-to-glow/

https://www.apa.org/ptsd-guideline/patients-and-families/cognitive-
behavioral

https://www.nami.org/

https://cpe.psychopen.eu/index.php/cpe/article/view/14351/14351.html

https://www.uclahealth.org/news/article/how-does-grief-affect-
your-body

https://positivereseteatontown.com/understanding-unresolved-grief/

https://www.mayoclinic.org/diseases-conditions/complicated-grief/symptoms-causes/syc-20360374

https:/https://www.news-medical.net/health/The-Health-Effects-of-Loss-and-Grief.aspx/www.news-medical.net/health/The-Health-Effects-of-Loss-and-Grief.aspx

Mindful.org

https://mhanational.org/resources/maintaining-boundaries-as-a-caregiver-go-from-guilt-to-glow/

https://athomeindependentliving.com/learning-to-say-no-as-a-caregiver/

https://mhanational.org/resources/maintaining-boundaries-as-a-caregiver-go-from-guilt-to-glow/

https://www.apa.org/ptsd-guideline/patients-and-families/cognitive-behavioral

https://www.nami.org/

REFERENCES

Academic and Clinical Sources

1. **Beck, A. T., & Emery, G. (1985).** *Anxiety Disorders and Phobias: A Cognitive Perspective.*
   - This foundational work by Aaron Beck (the founder of cognitive therapy) explains how cognitive distortions like catastrophizing contribute to anxiety and how reframing can correct these patterns.

2. **Burns, D. D. (1999).** *The Feeling Good Handbook.*
   - A widely respected book in cognitive-behavioral therapy (CBT), explaining cognitive distortions and how to reframe negative thoughts. Accessible for general readers but based on clinical CBT principles.

3. **Hofmann, S. G., Asnaani, A., Vonk, I. J., Sawyer, A. T., & Fang, A. (2012).** *The Efficacy of Cognitive Behavioral Therapy: A Review of Meta-analyses Cognitive Therapy and Research, 36(5),* 427–440. https://doi.org/10.1007/s10608-012-9476-1
   - This meta-analysis confirms the effectiveness of CBT techniques—including cognitive reframing—for treating anxiety and depression.

4. **Ellis, A. (1991).** *The Revised ABC's of Rational-Emotive Therapy (RET).*
    ○ Introduces the ABC model (Activating event, Belief, Consequence) central to cognitive reframing in Rational Emotive Behavior Therapy (REBT).

ABOUT THE AUTHOR

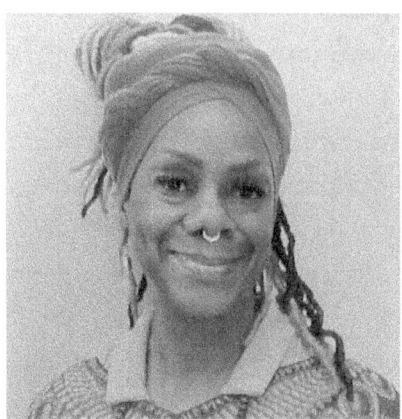

Terrie Larae Harris

Terrie LaRae Harris is a compassionate caregiver, insightful speaker, and dedicated community advocate, focusing on the profound journey of navigating grief and loss. Drawing from a deep understanding of the human spirit and her own lived experiences, she champions the integration of mindfulness and holistic wellness practices to support individuals through their healing process. Completed Biblical Studies from the International School of Ministries with a Diploma of Biblical Studies.

She is now a Spiritual Coach, devoted to guiding individuals on their journey toward healing, purpose, and divine alignment. Rooted in faith and driven by compassion, Terrie offers a safe, sacred space where people can explore their spiritual identity, overcome emotional barriers, and awaken to their inner truth.

With a background in ministry, human services, and personal life experiences that include overcoming grief, caregiving, and military service, her passion brings a unique blend of spiritual wisdom and real-life resilience, coaching is not about religion, but about restoration—helping people reconnect with God, rediscover their worth, and live intentionally with clarity, peace, and power, whether navigating a season of transition, seeking deeper meaning, or simply craving spiritual growth.

Terrie's foundational knowledge stems from her Bachelor of Arts in BTAS Human Services from Kent State University, which has informed her extensive work in the human services field. Including direct care and advocacy, she is a respected non-fiction writer. Her published work thoughtfully explores critical topics such as prolonged complicated grief, fostering well-being, and embracing personal growth while navigating the complexities of loss. Her writing serves as a powerful testament to her commitment to sharing insights and cultivating resilience in others.

At the core of Terrie LaRae Harris's work is a profound empathy for the human experience, her approach is characterized by unwavering compassion, a gentle yet firm commitment to empowering individuals, and a steadfast dedication to guiding them through life's most profound challenges with resilience and grace. She is passionately driven by the belief that even in the face of immense loss, individuals can discover renewed meaning and purpose in their lives and tap into the resilience to transmute pain into power.

Beyond her roles as a caregiver and writer, Terrie LaRae Harris is a dynamic force in her community. She actively engages in various thinking circles, serves on boards, and dedicates her time to Veterans services and hospitals. Her regular involvement in teaching, public speaking, and community initiatives underscores her holistic commitment to fostering healing and sharing vital information across all aspects of well-being, always with the goal of helping others navigate their grief journeys.

www.ingramcontent.com/pod-product-compliance
Lightning Source LLC
Chambersburg PA
CBHW061758120626
46550CB00005B/2039